Blue Eyeshadow Should Be *Illegal*

Paula Begoun

A BEAUTIFULLY DIFFERENT MAKEUP MANUAL

Revised 1986

Typography: Common Line Communications
Printing: Bookcrafters, Michigan

Copyright © 1985 by Paula Begoun
Beginning Press, 5247 South Dawson, Seattle, WA 98118
Second Edition: April 1986
1 2 3 4 5 6 7 8 9 10

ISBN 0-9615514-0-2

This book may be ordered directly from the publisher,
Beginning Press, 5247 South Dawson, Seattle, WA 98118
Please include $7.95 plus $1.50 postage and handling for each book ordered.

With Special Thanks

To David for bringing me closer to God and love; to Cheri for teaching me strength, commitment and editing; to Avis for helping me see into myself; to Grandmother for the joy of Sunday breakfast; to Richard for publishing his book first and if he could do it why not me? and to the first woman who did my makeup back in 1975 at the Marilyn Miglin Salon in Chicago.

Thank you all for helping me get to the point where I had a place to put this dedication.

Acknowledgements

Special professional thanks to: Photographer David Hagyard for his brilliant photography; Hair designer Emilio Davila from the Gary Bocz Salon in Seattle for his skill and talent; Jerry Kennedy for her patience; Stanford Poll for his generosity; Mary Sprague for her love and time; Common Line Communications' Michael, Barbara and Gary for staying calm in the face of type and camera deadlines; and Michael Esfeld and Steven Fleishman who would feel left out if I didn't mention them too.

Table of Contents

Table of Contents continued

Table of Contents continued

Why Call A Book, *"Blue Eyeshadow Should Be Illegal"*?

At first it was because I truly believed that it was a major mistake women frequently did with their makeup; over color their lids, letting the shadow or eye-pencil color be more noticeable than the eyes. In the long run though, I'm really easygoing. There are worse things than wearing blue eyeshadow (there's always bright lime-green or shiny rose-pink). Plus, everyone is entitled to their opinion, especially if they have reliable information and experience to base those ideas on. So *Blue Eyeshadow Should Be Illegal* became a title that would represent a different perspective on makeup and the cosmetic industry in general.

Of course, to be totally honest about the whole thing, *Blue Eyeshadow Should Be Illegal,* seemed a great title. Everyone, regardless of sex, age, income bracket, religion or ethnic background, reacted to it. The title became a great marketing tool. I figured women who wore blue eyeshadow would be interested because they would want to know how I came to such a ridiculous conclusion. Women who didn't wear blue eyeshadow would feel I knew what I was talking about. And because I never heard a man say, "Wow, I love when a woman wears blue eyeshadow," I thought, how could it fail?

This book is a compilation of what I have been teaching, reporting on and doing over the past ten years. It has worked for me and many, many others. I know you will find some, if not all of the contents, to be interesting and helpful. If nothing else, I promise it will be unique and fun.

Paula Begoun

The
Cosmetic
Connection

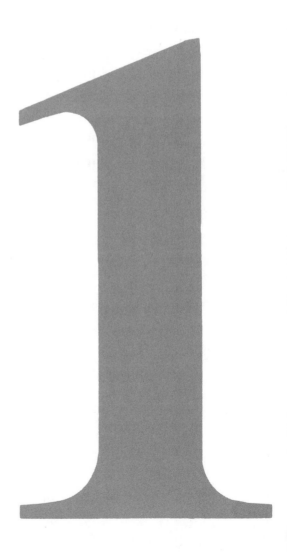

A Cosmetic Quiz — Test Your Beauty Frustration Level

I know, I know, who needs another beauty book? I understand your sentiments exactly. In my opinion if you were to take all the beauty books in the world and lay them end to end you should probably leave them there. So why, you're asking at this very moment, why do you need this one? It's a good question. Before you make any decisions, take the following test to see if you need the information in this particular beauty book. Get a pencil and paper ready and give yourself five points for each comment that applies to you. Good luck!

1. Do you think makeup can help you look more like the women in the magazines? However, no matter what you do or try you can't get your makeup to look like theirs?

2. You own one to five cosmetics that have never been used or used only once.

3. You own more than one blue eyeshadow and have noticed that no one on the cover of a magazine ever wears the stuff plastered all over their lid.

4. You purchased a cosmetic that looked different at home than in the store, or you just didn't like it the next day.

5. You have purchased an eyeshadow that shattered when you dropped it, the top of your foundation came loose and spilled makeup in your purse, or you have a blush compact or an eyeshadow compact held together with a rubber band.

6. You itched like crazy after using a cosmetic product or had an allergic reaction to a product in some way and felt helpless not knowing what you could do besides suffer.

7. You purchased a mascara that was labelled water soluble and found it wouldn't rinse off at all.

8. You came home from the store with a mascara that was labelled waterproof and found that it washed right off.

2

9. You purchased a lipstick or gloss which, via the lines around your lips, started moving its way to your chin or nose.

10. You bought an eyeliner pencil and when trying to sharpen it found that you needed to buy a special sharpener in order to use the pencil.

11. After buying the right sharpener you found that you eventually ended up whittling the pencil down to nearly nothing because the point kept breaking off, smushing away, disappearing or only one side would sharpen while the other retained the wood coating.

12. You felt a cosmetic salesperson lied, misled or gave you insufficient information about a product.

13. You don't understand the difference between a "drug" and a "cosmetic."

14. You enjoy the idea of glamour but don't want to take longer than 10 to 15 minutes to achieve it and most makeup routines seem to take at least 20 to 30 minutes.

15. You wonder why makeup has to cost more than steak or lobster.

16. You wonder why an ounce of foundation or a fourth of an ounce of shadow comes packaged in an enormous container and box that weighs a ton by comparison.

17. You bought a "wrinkle free" cream and discovered a year later you still had wrinkles.

18. You're skeptical and really don't believe that European aestheticians know anymore about skin care than their American counterparts.

19. You have wondered what face shape you have and then noticed everyone's face shape is supposed to be made up to look one way — oval.

20. You have read more than one beauty book and found it sounded just like the one you read before, you couldn't follow the techniques, or there was just too much information that you didn't want to do.

All done? Count up the points. If you scored between zero and thirty, you are either lucky or you don't wear makeup. Thirty-five to fifty points means you are one of the many who assumes that if you're patient and talk to another expert you'll find your dream-come-true cosmetic and be happy. Fifty-five or higher means that you want to scream at someone but don't know who. If you scored high and aren't upset, then you must have time and money to waste and it doesn't matter to you anyway. You can afford the eternal search for the perfect makeup product. But if you're one of the high scorers and can't afford to be or don't want to be, you've bought the right book. We're both upset and want to do something about the situation.

The expensive or complicated makeup and skin care routines touted by major cosmetic lines, fashion magazines and "beauty books" have reduced women's pocketbooks as well as their objectivity. Resisting media-induced ideas projected by a billion dollar industry is not easy. To be a smart consumer takes a lot of information and courage. (Information, inside this book, means practical and easy; courage refers to the capability of looking at the entire cosmetic issue from a new perspective.)

Blue Eyeshadow is not a book that will teach you how to mix eggwhites with avocados or oatmeal with honey to use on any part of the face to get it clean. *Blue Eyeshadow* will also not have you go through a lengthy cosmetic application of moisturizer, blemish cover, skin-color correcter, highlighter, foundation and powder, in order to start your makeup. If that's what you want, there are plenty of books offering just that, but not this one.

Who Can You Trust?

The only easily accessible information available to women, concerning the makeup industry, are articles in fashion magazines, such as *Glamour, Vogue, Bazaar* and *Cosmopolitan.* Although these magazines don't actually lie to the consumer about makeup and skin care, they don't give the reader the entire truth either. And when you think about it, they can't afford to.

Imagine you are the editor of a major fashion magazine. Congratulations! Now think about it for a minute. How can you permit articles to appear in your magazine that speak out against, or disparage a $750,000 a year or greater, advertising account? If that account says it can prevent wrinkles, are you going to publish articles that say, "in a pig's eye!"? Accounts such as this one are your bread and butter, your livelihood. You can't afford to publish a horde of negative articles aimed at the financial cornerstones of your business.

(The editor of a major magazine shared with me a story where one of the articles that ran explained how to give an inexpensive dinner party. The suggestion was to decant the expensive liquor bottles and pour in the inexpensive liquor. The result was that many of the major liquor advertisers threatened to cancel their ads for the remaining year if this kind of thing was going to continue. Needless to say, it did not continue.)

I wrote this book to provide an alternative to the one-sided information many women have inadvertently tumbled into concerning cosmetics. Makeup and skin care routines don't have to be exotic, scientific or natural to be good. With common sense, and a practical approach, no woman will have to ruin her budget, nor wonder "where the heck do I put this?" or "why can't my face look like those in the magazines?"

So who can you trust? Once you have looked objectively at the whole picture, in all its beautiful and beastly aspects; NO ONE BUT YOURSELF.

About The Author

Since your curiosity or interest has been maintained up to this point, I will take this opportunity to introduce myself and share with you who I am and how I developed my ideas and conclusions. I'm kind of wondering the same thing; at times, it even surprises me how this all came about.

At this writing, I am 32 years old and have been living in Seattle, Washington for the past seven years. Prior to and during that time, I was a successful makeup artist building a media-worthy resumé of celebrities I worked with, such as: Helen Gurley Brown; Lauren Bacall; Linda Lavin; Julia Child; and Chris Everett Lloyd to name a few.

In 1981, with a $700 loan from my father, (thanks Dad), and a concept that glamour didn't have to be expensive or complicated, I started a small cosmetic business that sold "no name" makeup, straight from the manufacturer. Three years later I had a partner and the business had expanded to four stores. In the spring of 1984 I sold all my shares of the business.

During that same period of time I lost 100 pounds, became single for the second time, had a local weekly radio spot, a national daily radio spot, aired a feature report on TV four times a week, played talk show guest across the country, and decided to change careers from makeup to Television Feature Reporter. (I see myself as a cross between Jane Pauly and Andy Rooney, except I'm not that blonde or short, but then again you can't be everything.)

In retrospect, the career of makeup artist mixed with consumer advocate and television reporter came about because 1. I was fairly good on television; 2. I could do my own makeup and anyone else's, quickly, simply and inexpensively; 3. after years of fighting acne, I discovered a skin care routine that, for the first time, showed me a light at the end of a bumpy (pun intended), frustrating trail and it only cost $10; 4. and after getting fired from two traditional makeup jobs in a row, it was a practical step to see if I could earn a living on my own, approaching makeup from a realistic non-hype point of view. (Truthfully and humbly, I really did get fired twice from traditional makeup-department-store-type jobs. Once because I was discovered encouraging a client to use my skin care routine of 3% peroxide and baking soda instead of the products that were being sold. The other time was for arguing with one of the Line Representatives in the store about the healing properties of a product. She told me to say it would heal the skin and I said I would do that if I knew which ingredients could perform that function. She said no one needed to know that and I disagreed. Guess who didn't come back the next day . . .)

In attempting to become this "Ralph Nader of Rouge" I chose to counteract the slanted advertisements and biased, misleading information that abounds in fashion magazines and "famous people" beauty books. There was no easy way women could gain access to reliable realistic information without resorting to technical journals. As a result, there was no way women could make educated decisions.

There was no one educating women that contouring the face to make it look different wasn't important or that astringents don't close pores, or that there aren't wrinkle free scientists up in the Swiss Alps, or that so-called European skin care routines or products won't make you any cleaner than American routines.

Being Realistic About Cosmetics

Lots of women have put their faces in the hands of salespersons (who often have limited information, experience and training), who emphatically assured them that their selections were wonderful and extremely necessary for their coloring and type of skin. Believing we purchased the basic requirements from someone "in the know", how often did we take those products home only to be disappointed or frustrated.

Influenced by the hope of beauty, many have bought the "perfect" foundation to compliment the new moisturizer which was made to be used with the pink toner with the blue cap. Sound familiar? Then you, as an unsuspecting, trusting customer, found that in the process of having used these wonderful, expensive commodities, that one or all of these products either didn't change a thing, irritated your face or was too much trouble. Of course, you figured it was your fault anyway because you should have bought the more expensive line two counters over. How can you stop this scenario from happening again? Read on.

7

To Correct or Not to Correct?

To start "debunking" some of the present day ideas promoted by major cosmetic lines it would be helpful to begin with a good fundamental working philosophy that can help you form a practical approach to makeup.

It is not necessary to apply makeup with the concept of doing a corrective makeup. In fact, the term "corrective makeup" offends me greatly. What is corrective makeup application? I'll explain by example . . .

A woman sits in the makeup chair and is asked by the artist how she would like her makeup done. She might respond, "Oh, any way you see me, it's up to you." More likely than not the artist will either think or say, "Let's start with a basic corrective makeup." Right? Not anymore.

Before and after ads encouraging corrective makeup remind me of the "old car needing a paint job" commercial. It starts out as a beat up Chevy before the new coat of paint and transforms into a brand new Lincoln afterwards.

There is an important fact you need to be aware of. With or without your makeup on, your face is fine. Yes, even without mascara, there is nothing that needs changing or altering about your face. I am frustrated with women going to cosmetic counters and being told that their skin is too pink and it should be more yellow, or that their skin is too yellow and should be more pink, or that their eyes are too far apart, or too close together, or too small, or too big, depending on who you happen to be talking to. I do not believe that women are inherently flawed creatures in need of cosmetics to be acceptable.

Makeup can be a fashion compliment to any woman's features and, like fashion, makeup is an alternative, not a necessity. The same way you wear jeans versus a dress depending on the occasion or your mood, choosing to wear or not to wear makeup is the same process. Any other attitude is limiting and overwhelmingly encourages a lack of self worth and esteem.

Now I know what some of you are saying, and it is perfectly acceptable and very dramatic to use "corrective" techniques in order to be altered for the camera or an evening look. (Corrective techniques involve things like changing the shape of the mouth, shading double chins, highlighting cheekbones or whiting out smile lines.) But in the mode of fashion makeup or street makeup, or makeup that will be seen in the light, too much makeup can be out of place. Effects that work for a camera can look silly and overdone when used on the street. In other words, a shading technique that singles a double chin tend to look like a shading technique that singles a double chin. (Makeup always looks like makeup, you're never really fooling anyone.) There are so many simple creative options available for women today that getting caught up on "corrective" is a waste of energy.

The path to a simple and attractive application (key word here: simple) is to define and color each feature as it exists without changing anything (or looking as if a can of paint hit you in the face). Whether it be casual, dramatic, business-oriented, glamorous, natural, daring, punk, sophisticated, preppy or whatever . . . it still can involve the same basic techniques. (Regardless of the style of blouse, there's only so many ways to button it). The idea that corrective makeup application is an everyday application strategy, is outdated and unnecessary.

Being Realistic About Yourself

It's no surprise to anyone that magazines and television create an illusionary world that can be misleading. Advertising campaigns often use pre-pubescent models or models that happen to be annoyingly perfect. These ads claim their products can make you look just like these adolescents.

Facts are facts, and neither childhood nor genetically inherited good skin can be bottled. No matter how hard we wish for it, there is no fountain of youth lurking at the bottom of makeup jars. (Though it is important to note here that makeup applied poorly or heavily can make you look older by making wrinkles show up more.)

Brand Name Addiction

Along with my feelings about corrective makeup and makeup addiction, is my strong belief that product loyalty doesn't make sense. The success of the major product lines in establishing that loyalty becomes apparent in how a woman responds to the question about what brand of makeup she is presently using. The answer usually reflects the amount of money that she has spent on said product. A customer usually whispers when she is using a bargain brand and if she's using the $25 a bottle brand you can hear her across the room.

It's so easy to fall into the cosmetic roller coaster rushing up and down counters of products lined with nothing but reams of advertising rhetoric, commercial jingles, media fables and promises. The reality about any particular makeup line is that they all have their good and bad points. The secret is knowing what those specifics are.

One secret is that the cost of makeup has nothing to do with whether a product works or not. I have used both inexpensive and expensive makeup which looks wonderful and is good for the skin, as well as expensive and inexpensive makeup that looked awful.

Advertising executives would lead us to believe that when we give our loyalties and money to a cosmetic line they are manufacturing our makeup for us. That isn't necessarily the case. What is really often happening?

Pretend you buy a brand name eyeshadow from two different companies. Did you know that these two eyeshadows could be absolutely the same eyeshadow? I mean *exactly* the same eye shadow? How? Simple. Both companies purchased it from the same manufacturer. What they do to the cosmetic after they purchase it is also relatively the same. They package it, distribute it, promote it and sell it. So you, the consumer, might pay anywhere from three to twelve dollars for the exact same eyeshadow, depending on whose name is on the package, bottle, or tube.

What I have just described is the reality of the cosmetic industry. It's called "farming out" your product line. It happens all the time, and in the long run, no matter who's making your makeup, the end results are that you could get stuck with a 500% − 2000% increase in what you pay for the final product if you buy according to packaging rather than contents. Price doesn't reflect anything about quality, how it will go on the skin, or how long the product you're considering will last. The only way to ascertain that information is to try the stuff on.

When women ask me what I think about a particular brand of cosmetics my response, regardless of the line, is always the same. All lines have products that are wonderful, mediocre, and awful. From the same counter, one blush or one lipstick might have just the perfect texture and the next one be grainy and dry. There are lots of reasons to account for the differences. One reason could be that their one lipstick came from a different manufacturing company than the other.

Why is it that your brand of cosmetics gets to be so expensive when compared to a less expensive brand that has been purchased from the same manufacturing company? In the final analysis price is determined by what that market will bear. If you're willing to pay $25 for a foundation and believe you'll look $25 better, they'll sell it to you for just that.

Hopefully your ideas of product line loyalties have changed. Don't take my word for it! Go to any library and check out a copy of *Drug and Cosmetic Industry* magazine and you can read about the manufacturing of cosmetics and cosmetic ingredients.

Think about it this way. Makeup is good, very good, when it works. Makeup is a waste of time when it doesn't work. That's not a difficult concept and it's what we're really talking about once we throw out the boxes, close the magazines and put the cosmetics on. It doesn't mattter whose name is on the package, what the ads say, or how expensive it is, if the makeup works and is good for your skin, then use it. You must be aware of all of these factors in the buying and use of cosmetics in today's high pressure, sales-oriented environment.

Advertising: Fact or Fiction

This is about the time you might be asking about truth in advertising; it's my favorite question. The Federal Trade Commission is the watchdog here and the cosmetic industry has cute ways of getting around the details of the guidelines. Cosmetic advertising is a prime example of the deceptive, manipulative use of the English language. It conveys an impression without actually substantiating anything at all. When they can't truthfully say a product will do something, they say that it can help do something. For example:

"Realistic help is here."

Well, what's realistic to you and what's realistic for the product is subjective and would never hold up in court. And the same applies to the word help.

"Works with the microcirculation of your skin."

"Works with" is always a good phrase, it doesn't mean a thing. Exactly what kind of "work" is it referring to? "Microcirculation"? Everyone has it near the surface of their skin, so a product sitting on top of the skin will touch "microcirculation". It won't change anything, but then that's not what the ad was talking about.

"Look younger, too."

Well, how much younger? Ten years or ten minutes. "Younger" is so vague, they could mean ten seconds.

"Replaces the fluids of youth."

We're mostly water, even youngsters are, so put some water in the jar and some oil so it stays on the skin for awhile and zap, you've replaced the "fluids of youth".

"The skin's ability for self-rejuvenation is helped."

Well that's the skin's ability not the product's, and help is that vague, means-nothing word again. Plus, all rejuvenation need refer to is what happens to a dried up dead leaf when you put

12

a little water and oil on it, suddenly it looks like a somewhat new leaf. But only temporarily; it hasn't been brought back to life.

"Medically tested."

You're never shown the test results nor is the lab or chemist mentioned. It can also be reworded to read "scientifically formulated", which does sound very scientific. Well, what product isn't scientifically formulated? The art of cosmetic advertising is vagueness, so read between the lines.

CAUTION: Before you read the following chapters, I'm concerned about a possible contradiction that you might find rather noticeable. At the same time that I'm warning you about the pseudo-information advertising rhetoric that is used dogmatically by cosmetic companies, I realize I also may sound somewhat dogmatic about my ideas and information. PLEASE UNDERSTAND THAT MY EMPHATIC PRESENTATION IS MY STYLE AND NOTHING MORE. Not that I don't totally believe what I'm saying and feel that the concepts are well presented and straight forward (without the intent to sell you anything except this book), but it is only information. Your role as consumer is to obtain enough credible information, and then make your buying decisions after you've weighed out the pros vs. cons and the facts vs. the fantasy.

Skin Care:
Or Now For Something
Completely Different

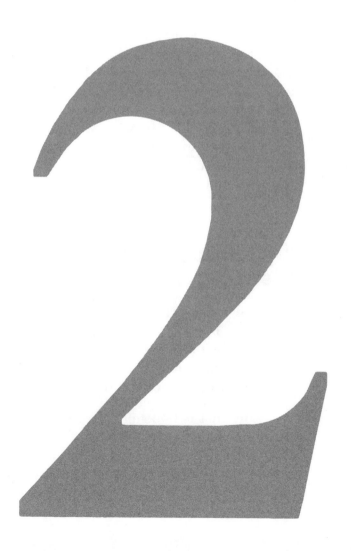

n this chapter we're going to discuss skin care: the myths and the facts. Among the "legends" handed down to women from everyone from friends and mothers to advertising executives and cosmetic experts, lay many half truths and a few not-so-white lies, not to mention many large prairie waffles.

I will shake up some long established beliefs about skin care routines that might surprise you. But first, let me mention something concerning your own personal skin care regimen: if it works, continue doing it.

If what you're doing now is successful, if you're pleased with your skin care routine, if you feel you aren't spending too much money and all the products make you happy, don't change. Just use this information as a new possibility to consider. I don't want anyone to use a new routine, mine, or anyone else's, unless they're dissatisfied and feel that their present process is unsatisfactory in some way. My ideas are an option, an alternative and a rather inexpensive alternative at that. My approach offers you a whole new concept in skin care. Since statistics show that every one to three years you will change your skin care routine and try something new, this is one to seriously consider.

First Things First. Let's Talk About Cleaning Your Face.

The most important thing to use whenever you clean your face is water. Why? Because we are water. Our cellular weight is 60-90% water and the environment is 75% water, there is nothing more natural than the use of water when cleaning your face, and nothing quite as inexpensive either!

Now that is hopefully the last time you will find me use the term "natural". *"Natural" and "good" are not synonymous words.* There are many things that are natural that I wouldn't recommend for your skin; urine, copper, radiation and formaldehyde are all "natural" but not necessarily good for your face.

16

"Natural" is one of the most overused and misleading advertising phrases on the market today. "Natural" doesn't tell you anything. It gives you no information. My advice is, ignore the word in any and all advertising claims.

If I'm not interested in natural, then why water? Aside from being inexpensive and plentiful, the most important factor about using water is that it is gentle to the face. **CAUTION:** WATER IS ONLY GENTLE IF IT IS TEPID WATER. Hot water burns and cold water shocks the skin. What makes this skin care process different from most others on the market is the theory that the skin doesn't have to hurt or even tingle a little to be clean. The major rule for all skin types is, if it feels uncomfortable once, don't do it again. Pain and cleanliness have nothing to do with each other.

Stress, Nerves and Irritation

The reason being gentle is so important to remember is because of the nerve endings' negative reaction to irritation. If I were to tell you your skin reacts badly to stress, most likely you would agree with me. Unfortunately it will react the exact same way to irritation. Nerves can't tell the difference between pain, stress, irritation or itching. To them it's the same thing. It follows that if stress is bad for the skin, so is irritation.

What physically happens when the nerve endings are triggered as a result of irritation? Nerves are attached to the skin, hair follicles, oil glands, veins (blood flow to the skin's surface), and the underlying structure of the skin. If you activate the nerve endings by irritation of any kind, the oil glands are going to produce oil, the skin can flake, and the blood circulation to the small veins near the surface of the skin will increase, which may cause capillaries to surge to the skin's surface. If capillaries are already present on your face, you'll make them redder. Do not stimulate any nerve endings if you can help it.

What I am concerned about is the expectation that you can have unblemished, soft, supple skin even though the skin is being abraded and irritated daily. There are plenty of irritants that bombard our skin all the time, some we cannot control, some we can.

Pollution is one common irritant that is bad for the skin, crazy work schedules and a frenzied home life are also awful. Extreme heat and cold are worse. It's difficult to control everything in our environment every moment, so let's control what we can, like water temperature, and be cautious about the external stress we subject our faces to.

Think Gentle

What I want you to consider now is, how you can be more gentle to your skin and how you can baby your nerve endings. Be gentle to your skin and it will do more than reward your face by looking good; it will feel good too.

How can we be more gentle to the skin? Here are the recommendations:

No bar soap! What soap is usually made of is lard and lye with other trace elements to give it smell, color, etc. There isn't much of a problem with lard as a substance that people put on their faces. Lard is a fairly innocuous substance that doesn't cause many problems for the skin. Although some studies on rabbits' ears show that it is possible that lard may accelerate blackheading and eczema. Also, be aware that even though soap when rinsed off may feel like it's completely gone, that the same soap film left in your tub or sink has easily been absorbed by the skin. The major problem and concern when using soap occurs from the effect lye has on our skin.

Lye, also called sodium hydroxide or potassium hydroxide, burns the skin. Soap hasn't really changed appreciably for years. We are washing with the same product that was invented centuries ago. This same bar of soap, this cake of lard and lye, when first invented was used maybe once a month or once every six months. Today we wash with it once, twice or more a day. It's possible we are burning our faces in the name of clean skin.

What most women believe is that the tight sensation they feel after using soap means their skin is clean. You know that feeling where if you open your mouth it pulls the skin around your eyes? If it's stretched taut it must be clean, because tight equals clean. The squeakier my skin the better off I am, right? What you're really feeling is irritated skin. Your skin and the nerves are probably in shock; that is why your face feels so tight and looks so red.

The only difficulty with asking someone to break a soap habit is that soap really cleans the skin beautifully. The issue is we do not need to burn our faces in order to be clean. The positive of being super clean doesn't outweigh the negative of burnt skin. Soap can drive your skin crazy. After washing with soap, if you have dry skin, you will have to run to your moisturizer and, if you have oily skin, the oil will resurface in about 90 seconds no matter how initially clean you feel; if you have combination skin, you will reinforce that dual condition. Do yourself and your skin a favor and consider giving up soap for cleaning your face.

No More Astringents

Free your face from fresheners, toners, astringents, and clarifying lotions or any other fancy-named tonics that are supposed to aid in cleaning your skin. (**NOTE:** *Some toners do not contain harsh ingredients, they are simply glycerin and water, which are fine for the face.*) In short, stay away from all products that contain alcohol in any form. The ingredient label lists alcohol content as "SD Alcohol" followed by a number. Also be wary of the cosmetics which say they do not contain alcohol. Quite often they have substituted something equally irritating, such as ammonia, formaldehyde (or a form of either), grapefruit or lemon. Yes, citrus in skin care products can irritate the skin due to high acidic content.

In all fairness though, toners and astringents do offer a way to remove excess cleanser and slough skin (remove extra skin cells that can block pores). Yet there are more gentle ways to deal with the problem of excess cleanser residue (like don't buy one that leaves a film behind: see section on cleansers) and sloughing the skin (see section on use of baking soda). But *astringents do not and won't ever close pores, they do not deep clean pores and they do not reduce oil,* if anything they make the skin oilier!

What's wrong with alcohol? It is a great disinfectant but only for surgical instruments that is, not skin. In order for an astringent to be a disinfectant, it needs to be 60-70% pure alcohol. When you purchase an astringent you're using mostly watered down alcohol, maybe some glycerin, borax, preservatives and coloring agents on the skin. You're not getting an effective disinfectant, though you are getting an effective irritant. (That tingly feeling is nothing more than irritation and remember what happens to the skin with any kind of irritation.)

More Gentle Thoughts

While you're tossing out your bottles of toners you might as well include facial scrubs and abrasives. These are the products that are advertised (along with those astringents) as being able to clean out pores. What little miracles could these products contain that would allow them to constructively get inside a pore and clean it out? These cleansers often contain tiny pieces of cement, fruit pits, seeds and other gritty abrasives or strong chemicals which are not going to clean out the inside of your pores. If you could get inside and clean pores out, as if you were a dentist drilling, you would be bleeding. Even if you manage not to bleed through all the pores you're cleaning out, you'll find that this stimulation of the nerves (attached to the oil glands) will simply produce more oil, thus refilling the pores. Now you have made the mythological deep pore cleansing situation worse. You're running your facial nerve endings in circles.

These little almond shells, and other abrasive cleaners, are also advertised as being able to slough off skin. The major problem with products designed for this process is: Who educated the peach pit to know the difference between a dead skin cell and a live skin cell, and how can it tell when a skin cell is ready or not ready to come off? The difficulty with these products is you can easily end up scrubbing more than is healthy for the skin. You end up burning the face or ripping it to shreds, and then, by following up with your favorite astringent, you burn it even more. The advertisements tell you this

20

process makes your face feel clean and fresh. I am sorry, but when you see red, that's inflammation, not clean. If you want to feel tingly fresh or look red and glowing, run up and down the stairs ten times. I promise you will not only look red, but you will have done something for your heart and lungs instead of just tearing up your skin! (**NOTE:** *Sloughing skin does have a place in skin care and I'll talk about that later, the present issue is one of degree.*)

This is a good time to clarify exactly what this "oil" is that the oil glands produce that causes so much havoc on the skin. The word "oil" is very misleading. For some reason, we assume that we actually have oil splashing around under our skin, like in mineral or olive oil bottles. That just isn't the case. The oil underneath our skin is hard. It is the same kind of waxy substance produced in our ears. This hard, whitish wax-like substance that is secreted by our oil glands explains why excess oil production stretches our pores and creates solid bumps when it gets over produced rather than just free flowing through.

Wax liquifies at surface temperature which explains the oil slick we sometimes experience on the surface of our skin. (Although in my case it's more like an oil tanker spill.) The black you see in a blackhead is not dirt, it is oxidized oil. The hard yellow-white wax that is in the pore meets the air and turns black. That's what a blackhead is. Don't be misled. A blackhead is not filled with dirt and astringents aren't going to get rid of it. Remember by using all these astringents and scrubs you over stimulate the nerves which react by activating the oil glands which in turn produce more wax which create more enlarged pores and potential blackheads. It's a real cosmetic merry-go-round. (**NOTE:** *A whitehead is much like a blackhead except it is oil trapped inside a pore that is covered over by skin and not open to the air which is why it stays white and does not turn black.*)

Hands Off

Simply put, DO NOT TOUCH YOUR FACE. This is one of the biggest mistakes that most women make and then blame the cosmetic industry for the results. First, hands rubbing over the face is irritating and, again, we already know what that nets. Plus, I can't tell you how often I've heard complaints about makeup that doesn't last through the day, or barely makes it out the door right after being applied. Most likely your makeup is not jumping off your cheeks and eyes. When you touch your face, rub your eyes, or rest your hand on you cheek, your makeup will end up on your fingers, or the palms of your hands, and not on your face.

Another thing to remember is that when you rest your head on your hand or rub your eyes you are pulling and dragging the skin which causes sagging. In fact, one way to make sagging worse is to clean your face by wiping makeup off with cold cream using a tissue or washcloth. Whether you wipe up, down or sideways, you help the aging process by rubbing, pulling, tugging, or, in any way, shape or form, moving the skin.

While we're on the unpleasant subject of sagging, the blunt reality is that wrinkles are affected by gravity and are not helped one little bit with facial exercise. Gravity ages the face like no other element, with perhaps the exception of the sun (which I will cover later in this chapter). Gravity is one of the reasons that wrinkles point downward and not up and facial exercises definitely aid that process. Notice the areas of the face that age first are the areas we use the most by smiling, puckering and squinting, which are exactly the facial contortions you're sup-posed to do when exercising the face. Now, I'm not encouraging anyone to stop using their face, but natural facial expressions are radically different from self-imposed ones. The only effect that stretching your face into all sorts of positions will have are; you will feel somewhat foolish and you will stretch out the elastin in those areas faster, thus causing your skin in those areas to sag even quicker. (Just what you need, right?)

Pretzel Logic

Before I get into the specific details of my skin care routine, let's examine what is really going on when following the recommendations of many major cosmetic companies. Product sequences can vary from company to company but the typical skin care routine goes something like this: (You'll recognize it immediately.)

First you wipe your makeup off with a cleanser which makes your face feel greasy. Following the cleanser, you're supposed to use an astringent to remove any remaining cleanser which makes the face feel dry. Now the problem of dry skin is met with the moisturizer which undoes the previous two steps. Finally, after you get your makeup on, you're told to powder the whole thing to undo the effect of the moisturizer. Now that you're not shining anymore (heaven forbid you should shine), you're sold irridescent eye shadows, irridescent blushes and shiny lip glosses (so your mouth can look like you're drooling) and you can shine all over again. Get the picture? It must be a plot. If not a plot, then definitely an absurd financial trap. Buying products formulated to undo the previous step is a trap. This average routine, including cold creams, day creams, night creams, night cleansers, toners or fresheners costs about $45 to $75. That doesn't even include scrubs, masks and other specialty items that can take the total to over $100.

The routine I use is an alternative to the expensive never-ending product purchase treadmill. My alternative and the products I recommend will cost you about $10 to $15.

What to do instead?

Five Easy Steps

STEP ONE: *Wash your face with a water soluble cleanser; one that rinses clean without the aid or use of a washcloth.* Most cosmetic lines have at least one. Use a water soluble cleanser that leaves your face feeling soft, instead of tight as if you had washed with soap and not greasy as when you use a cold cream. You should not feel the need to use an astringent to cut a greasy feeling on your face, nor need to run to your moisturizer to prevent oncoming dryness. Your face should feel clean and definitely soft. This cleanser should also remove your eye makeup without burning your eyes. Why remove eye makeup at the same time? Answer: So you don't have to use an extra product to wipe off your eye makeup which pulls the skin around the eyes and which simultaneously causes sagging. Also the cost of tissue you wipe with is exorbitant and irritating to the skin. When you use tissues your eyes and face go through the same irritation your nose does when you have a cold. The area around your eyes ages the fastest and is an extremely sensitive part of your face. It should definitely not be pulled, wiped, stretched or sagged in any way if you can possibly avoid it. Using a water soluble cleanser is also more time efficient. It gets everything done at the sink in one fell swoop.

There is a catch; not all water soluble cleansers are created equal. A good one should be a cross between a cold cream and a shampoo. A typical ingredient listing on this type of cleanser should contain (but not necessarily in this exact order): Water, mineral or vegetable oil, sodium lauryl sulphate, triethloamine, and should be fragrance free and contain no coloring agents.

Different cleansers for different skin types are not generally necessary. All skin types need to be cleaned gently and thoroughly. Oily skins and heavy makeup wearers can tolerate a slightly stronger cleanser that contains less oil. A drier skin can use a cleanser that has more oil.

Wondering how to choose between cleansers? Be aware that even though companies claim differences and on the surface they look different, inside the bottles they may be very similar. Besides checking the labels, you need to try the product before buying. You can usually convince most cosmetic sales-people to give you a small sample if you supply the container. (A container can be anything from a piece of tinfoil to a plastic bag.)

Upon examining several cleansers closely and familiarizing yourself with the words used on the ingredient label, you'll realize that their contents are not all that special or different.

One cleanser may claim to be made from totally "natural" ingredients and another one claims to be medically tested or scientifically formulated, which supposedly can do all these wonderful things for your complexion. Perhaps a dash of vitamins or eggplant or whatever has been tossed in for "good marketing" but the vitamins or food stated on the label do not necessarily reflect results. That's why it's important to try it before you buy it.

Something Completely Different For Acne

STEP TWO: *At night only, wherever you have blemishes, pimples, or clogged pores, gently massage a generous portion of baking soda over the blemished area and then thoroughly rinse.* Baking soda, when wet, turns into a slightly abrasive paste that when massaged over a whitehead or blemish can take off the top of the blemish. For the purpose of removing potential excess skin cells (sloughing) baking soda is great as an extra cleansing step once or twice a week.

Now calm down, I know that baking soda is abrasive and that I sound like I'm contradicting myself but let me explain. A certain amount of *gentle* sloughing action is good for the skin, especially if clogged pores are a problem or if you're a heavy makeup wearer. Plus, when you take a closer look at some specific characteristics about baking soda, you'll discover it's more gentle than you thought.

Why baking soda instead of other scrubs? For three reasons. First, because it is a fine, even-grained substance and as a result is less likely to scratch the skin. Second, baking soda is an anti-inflammatory agent. (When you get a bee sting you don't put honey and almond pits on it — but you would use a poultice of baking soda to reduce the swelling). Third and last, the soda action can break up the wax under the skin which caused the problem in the first place. For the money you won't find a product on the market that works any more effectively. (**WARNING:** YOU CAN OVERDO THE BAKING SODA. DO NOT OVER SCRUB.)

NOTE: *If the skin breaks out all over you can massage the baking soda all over the face, gently. Or you can use the baking soda with a little increased vigor over a particular blemish.* The benefit from this extra massage is to open the blemish up. The advantages of opening lesions are that you can more easily disinfect inside the lesion where the invading bacteria is present and it can also make "squeezing" easier. I'm not the first person who has suggested that you have to open a lesion and remove what's inside to get rid of it, but there are ways to do it that can help and ways to to do it that can damage. You can help by gently squeezing the surrounding skin with even pressure. If it does not give easily, leave it alone. Over squeezing damages the surrounding skin and can create ugly scabs and scars.

REMEMBER: Leaving the pimple alone is best when after a gentle massage with baking soda, gentle squeezing won't help. If the built up wax and fluid inside the blemish can be easily removed it is a great way to help promote healing.

STEP THREE: *Wherever you have blemishes, soak a cotton ball in 3% hydrogen peroxide and apply to the infected areas or areas that tend to break out* (be sure they're cotton and not some synthetic fascimile). You can buy 3% hydrogen peroxide at any drug store for a very low price. It is an extremely efficient gentle, disinfectant. 3% peroxide can easily be used in place of an astringent. Hydrogen peroxide unlike alcohol is an effective disinfectant at a 3% solution — 3% peroxide, 97% water. It does not burn or react on the skin where the skin has not been opened. (Alcohol burns the skin upon contact.) Plus, 3% peroxide with continual use can change the color of blackheading by turning it back to white. (It does this by reversing the oxidation process that caused it to turn black in the first place.) **CAUTION:** BE CAREFUL AS THE 3% PEROXIDE WILL ALSO LIGHTEN FACIAL HAIR AND THE SIDES OF YOUR HAIRLINE IF YOU GET IT WET WITH THE 3% SOLUTION. (Personally, I adore the inexpensive highlighting along my hairline. I tell people that I dye my hair and take care of my acne at the same time.)

In summary, 3% peroxide is inexpensive, gentle, a good disinfectant, changes the color of blackheads from black to white, can lighten the hairline and won't dry out the skin – not bad for 89¢. (**CAUTION: 3% PEROXIDE CAN BE DRYING FOR THOSE WITH ULTRA SENSITIVE SKIN, OR VERY DRY SKIN.**)

A question that I'm asked quite often concerning the 3% peroxide is, "If the 3% peroxide is so wonderful, why don't the cosmetic companies use it in their products?" A good question. The answer lies in the problem of product stability. Chemicals must remain stable or interact favorably with each other to make a cosmetic formula work. 3% hydrogen peroxide is a highly unstable ingredient. It can decompose upon contact with sunlight and air. That's why 3% hydrogen peroxide comes packaged in those little brown bottles and should be purchased in small quantities as it can break down very easily and become good old fashioned water. On the other hand, alcohol, and other common ingredients found in toners, can be mixed with practically anything and remain intact for long periods of time.

NOTE: *You can use 3% hydrogen peroxide as a preventative measure even when pimples are not present if you have the tendency to break out.*

You Want Me to Use Milk of Magnesia Where?

STEP FOUR: *For acne or oily skin the only facial mask I recommend is milk of magnesia.* I really do mean milk of magnesia. (In fact, I have a 64 ounce bottle of milk of magnesia on my makeup table, and not mint flavored either!) Milk of magnesia is liquid magnesium. What is liquid magnesium? It's a simple combination of magnesium powder and water that when mixed together becomes hydroxide magnesium which is a great disinfectant and absorbs oil, just what you need when dealing with acne. (I've been told that milk of magnesia is used in hospitals over bedsores to help heal them. That may be why it helps to heal acne lesions as well.) After cleansing, apply the milk of magnesia generously over the face. Leave on till dry, then rinse well, (or if you've had a spicy lunch, you can always lick your nose and feel better; just teasing).

When I first started my skin care routine for acne and oily skin, because mine was so severe, I used to wear milk of magnesia under my foundation every day. I would use just a very thin layer placed over the skin, when it dried I would place my foundation over it. I also used it at night as a facial mask and rinsed it off.

WARNING: FREQUENCY OF USE AND HOW LONG YOU CAN LEAVE THE MASK ON DEPENDS ON HOW OILY OR SENSITIVE THE SKIN IS. The more oil, the more often it can be used. The more sensitive, do not use all over or leave on for protracted periods of time. Never leave the milk of magnesia on overnight.

REMEMBER: The 3% hydrogen peroxide, baking soda and milk of magnesia are only to be used if you have a skin problem. If not, it is not necessary for you to include these products in your skin care routine. Don't treat what doesn't exist.

Facial Masks

For those of you who don't have oily problem skin and as a result aren't using the milk of magnesia, next time you set out to buy a facial mask, read your ingredient label, and don't be fooled by promises that clay or pieces of birch bark are going to do anything for you. Always read on the label where these "natural" wonders are listed; if they're not in the first four or five listings, you're lucky if you're applying one rose petal.

Then you should consider what those ingredients are doing for the face anyway. Truthfully, I have no idea what real positives come from most other masks. I only know what they can't do: **1.** You can't feed the face from the outside in (in other words, you can't put liver on your face and have lunch). The nutrients can't be absorbed into the skin without being broken down by the digestive system. **2.** Plants or minerals left on the face can prove to be irritating to a lot of sensitive faces. (Same can hold true for the milk of magnesia, it is best to rinse it off as soon as it dries or begins to feel even slightly uncomfortable.) Plus, for the little bit of food or nature in your mask there are a lot of preservatives added to keep the product from molding and creating a new life all of its own.

I have to admit that it is possible for facial masks to indeed clean and soften but there are no miracles, or cures, and definitely no freedom from wrinkles or acne by using them. They really provide no better results than what your daily skin care routine should be doing in the first place. Keep in mind that masks used once a month is much like dieting once a month.

Understanding Acne

To explain how 3% peroxide, baking soda, milk of magnesia and the theory of being gentle can affect blackheading and acne, it is helpful to understand how a pimple occurs.

One theory of why a pimple occurs is that the oil (wax) in the oil duct backs up and stretches the base of the oil gland under the skin. The duct swells beyond capacity and can break open. This means that the wax spreads over into the surrounding tissue and the skin becomes irritated. That creates further swelling and tenderness but not necessarily a complete pimple. What creates most pimples is when a bacteria called propiobacterium is present in the same duct that broke open. This bacteria interacts with the over-produced wax which, in turn, inflames the skin. This inflammation attracts white blood cells to the lesion in defense of this irritation and produces what we affectionately call a pimple. In other words, acne is really more of an over-reaction to our own oil production. The reason 3% hydrogen peroxide works is because it can kill this propiobacterium that is present without further damaging the skin or exciting more oil production. Milk of magnesia and baking soda can do the same as well

NOTE: *Many of the new over-the-counter remedies for acne contain 5% to 10% benzyl peroxide. To an extent this works the same as the 3% peroxide. The benzyl peroxide is much stronger and as a result, more irritating. Acne is already red and irritated; it would be nice for a change to do something for it that doesn't make it more red and irritated.*

In spite of all this explanation, please be aware that nothing gets rid of blackheads and acne entirely. Nothing except entirely calming down oil production, which can be done medically with Accutane (I'll explain that in a moment), or being gentle so the nerve endings can relax and reduce oil production.

By the way, one pimple does not make a case of acne. I can't tell you how many women I've talked to with one pimple on their chin who inform me they have an appointment with their dermatologist that week. That's truly over-reacting. What happens to skin sometimes, regardless of age, race, sex, diet, or religious preference, is that it breaks out and there isn't much a doctor, a cosmetic company, or the routine explained here can do to change that. Hopefully what steps 1 — 4 offer is a course of action you can take when you do break out.

Doctoring the Skin

Discussing dermatologists when it comes to acne is a loaded subject for me. What I have to say will most likely not result in my popularity with the medical profession.

Since the age of thirteen I've had varying degrees of exzema, acne and oily skin. It was awful. Over those formative years and into my twenties and now thirties, I thought my acne would be history along with my puberty; I'm still waiting. (If you're like me you always heard only teenagers break out. As I have endured the continued humiliation through the years, I now know and accept that when I'm ninety, under my wrinkles, there will be acne.) The truth is acne has little to do with age and a lot it seems to do with hormones. (Fact: As many menopausal women as teenagers may develop acne.) Between the ages of eleven and twenty-five I saw twenty different skin doctors who prescribed varying remedies that didn't work. With a medical history like that, is it any surprise I have strong emotional viewpoints on the effectiveness of dermatologists when it comes to acne?

I should mention that my experiences were before the days of "Accutane". Accutane is an oral drug that performs miracles for people with severe acne. Please discuss its use with your physician. Accutane is risky and not recommended for occasional acne.

The following are typical prescriptions you might receive for severe acne as well as one pimple on your chin:

1. Antibiotics: These may help control the acne in some cases, but one month later you'll probably have to go to your gynecologist for a vaginal infection. Not to mention your eventual adaptation to the drug so it can't be used again to fight other infections; it randomly kills good bacteria as well as bad.

2. Retin A: Has the tendency to make your face burn and itch.

3. Scrubs or abrasive pads: Resemble and feel like steel wool. (See section on Scrubs.)

4. Topical Antibiotics based in alcohol. (See section on Astringents.)

Generally speaking, the medical answer offered to acne victims is a routine that takes skin, which is already red and inflamed and makes it look more red and inflamed plus dry and flaky. To me that no longer makes sense.

That all brings back memories. As a young girl, I was carted back and forth from one dermatologist's office to another by my well-meaning family. I fondly remember one particular visit when my mother lit into the doctor for all she was worth. "If you can't help her, tell her! She'd rather know the truth! She washes her face eight times a day and does everything you tell her, and she still has acne!" No one ever told us that acne had nothing to do with how clean my skin was.

Even after all that, I do feel dermatologists are an option when it comes to severe acne, and some mild acne problems. It's a good idea not to expect miracles though if you choose to see one.

NOTE: *To help avoid or at least somewhat curb acne, be aware that any of the following can aggravate or cause acne:*

1. Allergies to milk fat or dairy products in general.

2. Problems with fluoride in toothpastes (especially if you just break out around the chin, check with your dentist and try brushing with baking soda for awhile and see what happens).

3. Irritation from your partner's beard (especially if you're just breaking out around the chin and mouth).

4. Not getting all your makeup off at night.

5. Allergies to shellfish or any other suspect foods or food groups (like yeast, sugar . . .).

6. Certain cosmetics, like foundations, moisturizers or cream blushes (especially if the lesions are occurring where you place the blush).

Test your sensitivity to those things by eliminating them one at a time and watching the results. It can make a marked difference.

Wrinkle-Free Creams and Scientists

STEP FIVE: *Moisturizing.* Wow, besides acne this is one of the most touchy, emotion packed, sensitive issues I can think of in skin care. I don't know what it is, maybe because we want to, we choose to believe the unbelievable. Most women, when it comes to their moisturizers are living in a fantasy world. Here's reality; there are *no* creams or lotions you can purchase or non-surgical facial treatments available that will change, alter, affect, prevent or decrease the wrinkling process one iota. (SUNSCREENS CAN PREVENT PREMATURE AGING FROM SUN EXPOSURE. See section on sunscreens, pg.37.) One more truth, and this one is the biggy, dryness and wrinkling are not associated, related, or involved with each other.

Stop shaking your head and I'll explain the confusion. The error in connecting dryness with wrinkles is that both appear on the surface of the skin. The similarities pretty much end there. Dry skin is caused by the inability of the surface layer of skin to bind moisture to itself. Wrinkling on the other hand, is purely a result of changes in the underlying skin or dermis and has nothing to do with what happens to the moisture or oil on the surface of the skin. Think about it. If wrinkles and dryness were connected, then ten year old kids with dry skin

32

would have wrinkles, but they don't. They wait till they grow up just like we do. Also, the opposite would be true. Women with oily skin would never wrinkle, and I can attest they do.

Wrinkling is the primary evidence of the aging process and is primarily related to that. If you could stop the aging process, you could stop wrinkling. We can't do the former, so the latter is impossible too. Regardless of the touted ingredient, no matter how medically wonderful it sounds, it's just not possible to stop wrinkles via cosmetic products. Even if these products could stop the wrinkling process or change the skin, the product would no longer be a cosmetic. It would, under the FDA guidelines, become a drug (the difference is discussed later in this chapter).

Now that I've pulled the "wrinkle-free" rug out from under you, let me make my way back into your good graces by mentioning two things that can change the appearance of wrinkles, namely collagen injections and facelifts. A wrinkle occurs because the collagen (support tissue) of the skin breaks down. Collagen injections (not collagen creams), temporarily build up the skin's depleted supply. Violà, for six to eighteen months no wrinkles, and then you go for another injection and repeat the process. Facelifts and eyetucks are involved surgical procedures which simply cut away the sagged skin.

My mostly sincere recommendation: Take all the money you will ever spend on wrinkle creams and put it in the bank. Then by the time you're in the market for tucks, lifts or injections, the money will be there with interest.

You think we would have learned our lesson after we bought hormone creams advertised as preventing wrinkles, and despite this, we still got wrinkles. We just don't learn. We want to believe that there are secret laboratories somewhere in the Swiss Alps with wrinkle-free scientists who have packaged the fountain of youth for only $400 a pound (that's $25 an ounce).

I can hear you asking, "So, what can moisturizers do?" Moisturizers can benefit the skin by counteracting evaporation and helping to bind water to the skin cell. It does this by supplying your skin with additional oils that your oil glands may not be providing for you.

No matter what you do cosmetically to your skin, (except for the obvious things like rubbing and pulling) you have little or no control over the inevitable wrinkle. *The inevitable is already determined by your parents, your health, your diet, your environment, your suntanning habits and the effects of gravity on your skin.* What you are capable of doing for the skin is reducing superficial dryness. If the skin is dry, a moisturizer simply makes the surface of the skin look smoother and softer temporarily. In short, the fact of being born female and being over the age of 21 does not automatically mean you need a moisturizer. You *do* need a moisturizer for dry skin but don't buy someone else's oil when your skin produces enough of it's own. Oily skin doesn't need a moisturizer as it has its own built in.

Reading Between the Lines

The cosmetic industry takes full advantage of the fear of aging. Their ads allude that their products can possibly alter the "signs" of aging or "replace lost fluids." Don't those words sound meaningful? "Fluids" and "signs"? Actually "fluids" refer to either water or oils because that's what our skin is predominantly composed of; water, and the surface is covered with oil. The "sign" of aging is probably dryness, and almost any moisturizer can help that. So truth-in-advertising again is cleverly avoided. Please read your ingredient labels and if you're not finding at least two or more oils in the first five ingredients, you're buying a lot of water and wax and you need the oils, not the wax.

The two oils can be either a mineral oil and a vegetable oil or a mineral oil and an animal fat. The mineral oil stays primarily on the surface of the skin and prevents dehydration by keeping air off the face. Animal or vegetable oil absorbs into the skin and protects the lower surface layers of skin.

NOTE: *Mineral oil by itself can be dehydrating.*

Specialty moisturizers, such as eye creams, throat creams, and night creams are usually just extra oil and wax. Using almost any form of pure oil can replace a specialty cream. So, economically speaking, you can skip the extra waxes in the fancy creams and just use the oil. Simply use your daytime moisturizer at night and place the oil over the drier areas around the eyes, cracks at the side of the nose, wherever. If you don't have areas that are more dry than others, then you can forget this extra step all together. And it doesn't help to put anything over the lines, but if it makes you feel better, it won't hurt. (Like the old joke about the chicken soup: An older woman attending a funeral interrupts the eulogy by yelling out, "Give him some chicken soup!" The Rabbi replies, "Madame, it wouldn't help." The woman says, "It couldn't hurt!")

NOTE: *No woman needs more than one reliable moisturizer regardless of the time of day or night she chooses to wear it.*

What's in that Stuff?

As stated previously, when you buy a moisturizer you are buying someone else's oil to replace what your skin doesn't have. Indeed, that is exactly what most moisturizing creams are: 60% to 90% water and oil.

Now here's a good question. If most moisturizing creams are oil and water, why don't they look like oil and water? Answer: It's the wax-like thickeners they add to a product which turns it into a moisturizer's traditional form. The exclusive formulas you're rubbing into your face are comprised of water, oil, wax, some preservatives, coloring and a touch of fragrance, including the latest miracle like placenta, collagen, or elastin.

Whether the water is purified, extracted from some plant such as aloe, or is distilled, it is still just water. The same is true for the oil component, be it olive, shark (squalane), peanut, sesame, coconut, Wesson, almond, cod liver or Vitamin E, it's still just oil once inside the jar.

Waxes come in several forms; synthetic, such as by-products from the manufacturers of soap, or "natural", such as beeswax or tallow. Again, wax is wax. Typically, an agent to help blending and movability is added and there's the occasional anti-freeze to keep the cream from changing in varying temperatures, plus the latest fad from some science lab somewhere, and, voilà, you have moisturizer.

NOTE: *Collagen as a cosmetic ingredient placed in creams, works the same as lanolin and mineral oil do in a product. It binds moisture to the skin, but no better and no worse.*

Forget Skin Type?!

If you're wondering why I haven't discussed skin type, it's because I think it is misleading and confusing. The discussion of skin type tends to dwell on solving a problem that is based on some media constructed concept of what normal or flawless skin is supposed to be. Yet the idea of normal skin is unrealistic and ignores the dynamics and ever-changing status of our skin. And if we define normal as what is most common amongst most people, then skin with problems would be normal, and skin without problems would be abnormal.

The secret to good skin care is to listen to your skin. Skin is not independent from the weather, your diet, your emotions, or your skin care habits. If you wash everyday with a bar soap and then follow up with an astringent and then moisturizer, you should not be surprised when you discover combination skin (dry and oily).

Treating the skin gently, not drying it up and then greasing it back up, is one way to prevent dual skin problems; avoiding hot and cold water is another; using heavy wax laden creams which can clog pores is another, and using a moisturizer when you have your own oil is still another. Listen to your skin and deal with what is needed. For example: If your skin is oily you may need to go over your face with the cleanser twice, not just once.

REMINDER: Take care of what you see, not what you fear.

Of course skin type does exist, but it changes, depending on the many factors we've been discussing. The advertising gimmick of normal skin is a frustrating myth that is more like the proverbial carrot in front of the horse. In that passionate search to achieve perfect skin we end up doing and spending too much.

One More Time: The Sun

A word on the sun and your skin. Even though it's boring and you've heard it a thousand times before, one more time won't kill you. Sunshine directly on bare flesh ages the skin, dries the outer layer, thickens the skin, breaks down skin fibers and is generally worse for human skin than almost any other element in our environment (with the exception of gravity and Chicago in the winter, which we can do nothing about).

Suntanning ads would have you think otherwise, but then they're trying to sell tanning oils, aren't they? A very practical, although deadly dull idea, is to avoid exposing your skin, especially your face, to direct sunlight. If you simply cannot avoid being in direct sunlight without a hat or cover-up of some kind, use a good sunscreen containing PABA (there are plenty on the market) and continue reapplying every few hours. SUNSCREENS DO NOT LAST ALL DAY. THEIR EFFECT WEARS OFF WITHIN A FEW HOURS. Also be sure to reapply your sunscreen immediately after swimming or exercising.

My firm advice to all women who really want to do something about the aging process is to stay out of the sun, don't pull on the skin and stop worrying about growing up. You will look younger longer if you do.

SUGGESTION: If outdoor sports and athletics is the way you spend time, especially cold weather sports, including running, be sure to carry a tube of chapstick or clear lipstick that contains a strong sunscreen. This is a convenient, easy way to glide protection over the face at anytime you need it. Plus the consistency and ingredients in the chapstick and lipstick are great at protecting the face from the wind as well as the sun.

A Few Quick Comments That I Haven't Mentioned

Hypoallergenic

There is no such thing as hypoallergenic — it's a scientific sounding word with no legal basis. Calling a product "George" has just as much meaning if not more; at least you might know who George is. What you are allergic to is specific to you and there's no way a product can know that ahead of time.

Many allergic reactions are caused from a combination of products: Your foundation mixed with an eyeshadow, or a moisturizer worn under a new blush. It isn't always one specific thing and to make matters more complicated, emotions play a part too. Your moisturizer and the fight you had with your mother could trigger a reaction.

A typical allergic reaction can come from sleeping while still wearing your makeup. Makeup left on overnight is a powerful irritant to the surface of the skin. Next time you wake up in the morning with half your face on and half your face on the pillow, it won't be such a mystery what caused your eyes to swell and itch or your face to break out.

If you are convinced that you did have an allergic reaction to a product, return it. Most companies will refund your money. Besides they should be informed of products that may be causing problems for the population as a whole. If you don't inform them, they won't know.

Drug vs. Cosmetic?

Federal legislation distinguishes a drug as "articles for use in the diagnosis, cure, mitigation, treatment or province of disease or intended to affect a structure of the body."* Cosmetics are described as "articles for use intended to be paired, sprinkled, or sprayed on or introduced into or otherwise applied to the body for cleaning, beautifying, promoting attractiveness or altering the appearance."* In this country, drugs are stringently

*Taken from the Code of Federal Regulations #21 – Parts 600-700.

controlled, cosmetics are controlled as much as tea. Knowing that, would you really want something that had little or no guidelines (involved in its formulation) to absorb into your skin and change it?

Positive Attitude

There are worse things than oily skin and wrinkles.

H_2O_3

3% hydrogen peroxide will burn slightly on contact with open skin. That's okay, but if it burns a lot dab off the excess. **REMEMBER:** Skin care should not be painful.

Hair

Hair, whether it be on our head or any other part of the human anatomy can pose problems. On the head it's usually not having enough and on the body it's usually having too much. Excess body hair can be taken care of in one of five ways; shaving, tweezing, waxing, bleaching (lightening the hair) and electrolysis.

Shaving is inexpensive, easy and great for large areas like the legs. For the face though, growback begins in less than eight hours and a five o'clock shadow on any woman is never desirable.

Tweezing is great for small areas like eyebrows, but for larger areas it is time consuming and because of variable hair growth, can be a painful everyday procedure.

Waxing is much like tweezing in that the hair is being yanked out close to the root. The difference is speed, waxing is fast, it gets lots of hair all at once. The growback for waxing and tweezing is about the same. The negative part of waxing is that you have to wait for the hair to grow back in and obtain some length before you can wax again.

Bleaching is excellent for small areas and I prefer it to waxing and tweezing for facial hair. There is no growback or stubble, and it's inexpensive. The only negative is that many of the products available on the market turn the hair yellow and yellow facial hair is not necessarily any better than black. A good bleach recipe to use to turn the hair white is the following:

1   Teaspoon Lady Clairol Instant Whip
2   Teaspoons Clairoxide Developer
      (20 volume peroxide).
5   Pinches Lady Clairol Lightening Booster
      (comes in a small red and white package).

Mix together. Apply to hair with cotton swab. Wait ten minutes. Rinse off with cool water.

Electrolysis is wonderful for truly unwanted hair that won't change fashion (like moustaches). The problem with electrolysis is that it's expensive, time consuming and depending on the technician who performs the procedure, it can be a waste of time. Be sure to check out the credentials and obtain personal recommendations if you opt for this procedure.

In Summary, Here is My Skin Care Guide:

1. Twice a day wash with a water soluble cleanser. AVOID BAR SOAP. The cleanser should remove your eye makeup at the same time. Use tepid water — hot water burns and irritates, cold water shocks and irritates.

2. If you have blemishes, at night only, while the face is wet, massage blemishes with baking soda. Rinse well. Dry face gently. (Be careful; you can overdo the baking soda.)

3. Twice a day soak blemishes with 3% hydrogen peroxide. Let dry.

4. For blemishes, as a facial mask, use plain milk of magnesia. It acts as a disinfectant and absorbs oil. **NOTE:** *If you're not breaking out, if you don't have blackheads, then you don't need to use the peroxide, baking soda or milk of magnesia.* If you do have dry skin and still break out, use the baking soda, milk of magnesia and peroxide over the lesions only.

5. If your skin is dry, moisturize at night by spraying the face with a light mist of water and then spread the moisturizer over the water, let it absorb and dab off the excess. Do not rub or massage anything into your skin. Wear a moisturizer in the daytime if necessary. Moisturize when out in the sun with a sunscreen containing PABA. (As of March 1980, any lotion containing 5% or more solution of PABA can be labelled as follows: "This product reduces the carcinogenic effects of the sun and retards premature aging.") USE A PABA SUNSCREEN AND REAPPLY WHEN SITTING OUT FOR MORE THAN TWO OR THREE HOURS AND IMMEDIATELY AFTER SWIMMING AND EXERCISING.

6. At night, after your moisturizer has absorbed, pure lanolin, pure Vitamin E oil or any pure oil can be used over lines, around eyes or over dry patches instead of expensive eye creams, which generally contain the same ingredients. Read your ingredient labels.

7. Never use alcohol on your face. That includes all astringents, toners and fresheners. Alcohol's effect on the skin is dehydrating.

8. Remember that gravity plays a large part in the aging process. Don't help gravity do its job of pulling at the skin by wiping off your makeup.

There it is. Even if you're skeptical . . . my skin care routine is so inexpensive it's worth giving it a chance. I've been doing it now for over six years and my skin clears up when I just think of all the money I've saved.

IMPORTANT RECOMMENDATION:
Cleanser: Cetaphil (available in most drug stores).
Moisturizer: Lubriderm (available in most drug stores).

Blue Eyeshadow
Should Be Illegal:
An Owner's Manual

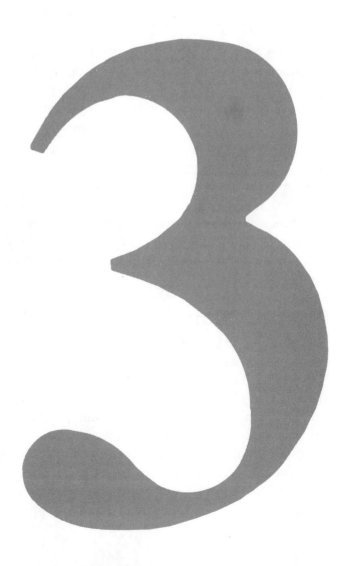

I t has never been recorded in history that anyone has ever dropped dead from modern makeup. Yes, there have been abused rabbits, and there are products with harsh ingredients and potential negative side effects. Yet we are still walking and talking and, most of the time, looking relatively attractive.

Makeup is remarkable. Modern cosmetic science, regardless of my frustration, should be congratulated. They have devised products that impart color to the skin, stays there for hours, does not melt in the interior of a car on a hot day or freeze when left in an unheated house in Chicago during the winter, and above all does not grow strange molds or fungus despite the fact they will spend most of their lives in a hot damp bathroom.

The truth of it is, makeup can produce minor miracles and major problems. In other words, makeup at its best can make you look great, or at its worse, make you look awful. And, if you'll forgive me for being repetitious, price has nothing to do with how you look . . . education does.

With that in mind, this next section explains my basic makeup application techniques and theories. As a makeup artist, TV-reporter and a woman who definitely enjoys wearing makeup, my priorities are to be sure I look good, without wasting time. If you're curious about the way my makeup appears on the cover of this book, and would like to learn how to do it yourself , the step by step formula and decision process is what follows.

Preparation

Because makeup goes on poorly over unclean skin, it goes without saying — even though it's been said a million times before, the first step in proper makeup application is to always have a clean face. After washing your face with a water soluble cleanser, apply your favorite moisturizer, but only if your skin is exceedingly dry. Under a foundation you do not need a moisturizer if your skin is not dry. Many foundations contain the same ingredients as your moisturizer does, so it isn't necessary to double up products. It makes more sense not to bother with a moisturizer. Never do more than you have to!

You may have been told that a moisturizer will protect your skin from the foundation but that's not possible. Moisturizers are made to absorb into the skin and once they do, for all intents and purposes, they're gone and they can't prevent anything else you put on from going where it wants. In addition, you wouldn't want a moisturizer that creates the type of occlusive barrier necessary to perform that function of protection for lots of reasons: It would feel and look either like an oil slick or a layer of wax; it would be heavy and you would probably then be told you need something under it to protect your skin from such heavy protection.

If you feel a moisturizer helps you get your foundation on better, there could be a problem in your application technique or the type of foundation you're using which are discussed in the next sections.

Speaking of doubling up products; special eyelid foundations, blemish covers and color correctors for skin tone are completely unnecessary. They complicate an otherwise simple process of starting your makeup:

Special eyelid foundations are usually very similar to regular face foundations. These two so-called "different" products can be almost the same thing packaged in different containers. Using your foundation on the eyelid will perform the same function this special lid foundation is supposed to do.

Blemish covers, if they don't match the foundation exactly, will show as a different color over the area. Or, if it is the same color it will place too much product over the lesion, bringing attention to the very problem you were trying to hide. Your foundation is more than sufficient to do the job of covering the redness.

Color correctors (those bottles of pink, lavender or yellow, meant to be worn under the foundation to alter skin color) are very similar to moisturizers and have little to no effect after they absorb. Consider the results if they did have an effect. The color of the corrector would mix with the foundation and you would end up with a very strange shade of foundation. Besides, what's wrong with your skin color in the first place?!

It's hard for me to imagine that anyone really believes they need, or want, to wear a moisturizer, color corrector, foundation, eyelid foundation and blemish cover just to get the face ready for blush and eyeshadows!

Highlighting

Most makeup routines start the same way; you begin the process by using a white, near white, or very light fleshtone highlighter placed at the inside corner of the eyes, but only if this area isn't already light by itself. If the under eye area is naturally white, like a goggle effect, it may actually be necessary to apply a deeper color (like fleshtone or slightly darker than fleshtone) under the eye to reduce that separation.

Highlighters come in several different forms. My favorite highlighters are creams; sticks tend to be dry and pull too much on the face and liquids have too much movement so they tend to be hard to control and smear easily, providing very little coverage. Creams on the other hand, are in a form that is ready to use. They are the right consistency and texture and work well with a liquid foundation. In addition, because the product is a cream, it tends to contain the same ingredients as a moisturizer, so it is still not necessary to double up products.

The application of this white highlighter cream will offset the natural shadows occurring in the eye hollow itself. The logic for using white, or as close to white as you can get, is like highschool "Art 101." When you need to make dark paint lighter, you wouldn't use blue, yellow or fleshtone to make it lighter; you would use white. Especially when you wear a foundation, this white is essential as foundation alone will not work to make anything lighter. To be sure there are no edges, it is essential the foundation blends over the highlighter making the combination appear lighter under the eye. A fleshtone highlighter in this area will mix with the color of your foundation and you'll simply end up with a third color which will not necessarily be any lighter, only different.

NOTE: *Fleshtone highlighters are perfect when used without a foundation. Place the color under the eye and blend out the edges slightly toward the temple and on to the cheek.*

When working with a white highlighter and foundation, do not place the highlighter all the way under the eye in a half-circle, or on the eyelid (unless the eyelid is also dark). Placing the white all the way around the eye can create a raccoon mask. (Raccoon eyes, no matter how nicely applied and blended, are definitely out!)

Depending on the length of your nails (when nails are long you can hurt yourself), use your finger or dampen a cotton swab (to control the fuzzies) and place the white highlighter in a half-inch crescent starting at the corner of the eye (called the tear drop) moving towards the center, covering one third of the area under the eye.

Wait — do not do any blending just yet. For the sake of time and final results, wait until the foundation is placed on the face and then do your blending.

NOTE: *It is often recommended to use the highlighter over age lines to make them less apparent (which I think looks more obvious because of the extra layer of makeup it requires), or over the center of the nose, top of the cheekbone, chin and other areas for accent and enhancement. That is*

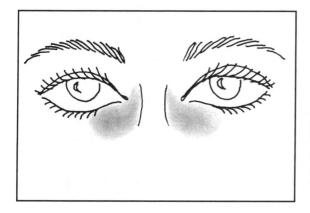

A) CONCEALER

Place white concealer on with the index finger or cotton swab hugging the inside corner of the under eye area.

indeed an option, but one that is complicated and time consuming, even for women adept at makeup. Plus you can net the same results by applying the rest of the makeup correctly. (I've used none of those techniques on my makeup as it appears on the cover and all those areas look highlighted.)

Foundation

Why foundation at all? To assure that everything else goes on evenly. Foundation is applied to those areas where other powdered colors, such as blushes and eyeshadows, will be placed. Foundation gives the rest of the makeup something to hold on to, since skin, all by itself has no adhesive properties. Blushes and eyeshadows have some ability to cling, but mostly they have more in common with baby powder. Ever put powder on after showering? Where's most of the powder? Right; on the floor. Applying foundation is essential, and the more evenly applied, the better everything else will go on as well.

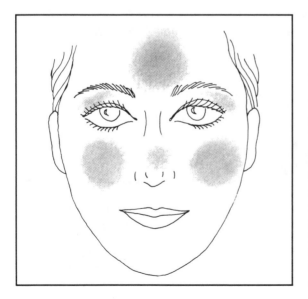

B) FOUNDATION
With a sponge, apply foundation generously to the central area of the face only, concentrating on the upper ⅔. Then blend with a dry sponge in a down and outward motion. Always avoid placing color near the jaw. Over the eye, fold sponge in half and dab foundation in place.

Sponges

The best application technique when applying foundation is to use a flat, quarter-inch thick sponge without holes. This shape and density provides the smoothest application possible. Using a cotton ball or cotton pad deposits tiny pieces of itself all over your face, and ends up wiping more foundation off, than on. Using your fingers will streak and blend the makeup unevenly. (Imagine finger painting walls. Using your fingers on your face will net the same appearance.) Also, fingers rub perspiration into the skin which is irritating. Ever get perspiration in your eyes?

The thick wedge sponges that you find available at many cosmetic counters are difficult and clumsy to use. They crumble after a few uses; they're hard to wash; they drag over the skin; and, because they are so thick, most of the foundation absorbs deep into the sponge where it can't be used. That can waste a lot of product. Wedge sponges are used primarily in theater and TV for pancake makeup, not everyday liquid foundations.

NOTE: *The sponge is a wonderful blending tool to keep nearby at all times. When softening edges of blush or shadows, work with the side of the sponge that you used to spread the foundation with over the face. This will allow the sponge to glide over the face instead of dragging, which can tend to streak the makeup.*

Blending

Using your nice flat square sponge, place the foundation generously over the central area of the face. The foundation goes on in large patches over the highlighter, the eyelids, cheeks and forehead but only in the center. Avoid placing lots of dots all over the face which can cause too much foundation to be blended into the edges where you need less than you do over the center. (See diagram B)

Hold the sponge between the first three fingers and thumb. Spread the foundation down and out over the entire face (still avoiding the eye area) in the direction of hair growth, with a stroking, buffing motion. Blend the foundation color from the center into the perimeters of the face, leaving no line of demarcation at the jaw or hairline. When blending the foundation, do not try to force it into the skin. There is a fine line between blending something on and wiping something off. Instead, blend a thin layer over the face smoothly with your sponge. Use the edge of the sponge without foundation to remove any excess foundation that tends to occur under the eye, and at the hair and jawline.

Once the foundation is blended over the face, now you can finally blend the white highlighter together with the foundation, out under the eye, by dabbing, not wiping, with the sponge. Saving the highlighter for last prevents blending it onto areas you don't want to it to go.

WARNING: NEVER EVER PUT MAKEUP OF ANY KIND ON THE NECK. There is nothing quite as unattractive as a collar with makeup on it. The foundation should match the skin so exactly that you only need to blend down to an inch above the jawline to insure that a turn of the head doesn't rub makeup onto your collar.

CAUTION: THERE ARE PLACES ON THE FACE YOU WILL BE LIKELY TO MISS WITH FOUNDATION THAT NEED TO BE CHECKED. These are the "corners" of the nose, the tip of the nose, the corners of the eye (especially over the highlighter), and the edge along the lower eyelashes. There are also places that you will "hit" with the foundation that you should avoid. These are the ears, the jawline and the hairline, (especially on blondes). Be careful to remove this excess if you've gone past your mark.

Mini-Application

If you hate the feel of foundation, don't worry. You needn't apply it all over the face. Remember, foundation is only really needed to give the blush and shadows something to adhere to. When the foundation color matches the face exactly (and after you finish this section, it will), you can apply a "mini-application" of foundation over those areas where the other colors will be placed. This way you won't feel heavily made-up and the blush and eyeshadows will still go on evenly.

To apply a mini-application, start with the highlighter as you would for a full application. Then place the foundation over a mask-like area between the eyes and mouth including the nose and cheeks. There is no foundation coverage needed on the chin or forehead. Be sure to blend the edges carefully with your sponge.

Matching Skin Color

Keep in mind that skin and foundation color should match exactly. If you are pale, accept the fact that you are pale and buy a foundation to match, not to darken. That you have a foundation on at all, should be one of those things only your makeup artist knows for sure. Choosing a foundation shouldn't be all that complicated, yet it is one of the more confusing aspects of makeup application. One of the problems of matching skintone is understanding what "skintone" means.

Traditional names associated with skin color are: Olive, when the skin appears ashy or green grey; sallow, when the skin takes on a yellow or golden shade; and ruddy, when the skin has shades of pink or red. Unfortunately this information can be misleading. If your skin is ashy are you going to choose an ashy foundation? Or if your face is very red are you going to buy a red foundation? To aid your purchase of a foundation, understand that what you want to identify is your underlying skintone which, most always means, you are dealing with varying yellow-brown tones. The coloring agent of the skin is melanin, which is brown. The yellow comes from the carotene in the skin. Carotene is the same substance you find in such foods as zucchini and carrots. In fact, if you eat enough foods containing carotene, your skin will take on a definite yellow cast. The amount of melanin mixed with the carotene in your skin determines your skin color.

The pink appearance in the skin can come from many different sources: Circulation in the tiny blood vessels found close to the suface of the skin; broken capillaries (that look like tiny red lines on the face); sunburn; skin irritation and acne. Next time you purchase a foundation, stay away from the pinks and rose tones that over-color the face and, because it is so different from actual skintone, becomes too obvious. Choose a realistic color that will give you the best results. The color you're looking for is best described as a shade of yellow beige, yellow porcelain, yellow tan, etc. (Foundation is not meant to "color" the skin; that's what blush, lipstick, and shadows are meant to do. It's meant to create an even neutral base for the makeup to be applied to.)

A Foundation Trick

Although you are attempting to match the skin tone exactly, in theory you are really matching the foundation to the neck. If the face is darker than the neck and you put on a foundation that matches the face it will look like a mask because of the difference in color between the two. The rule for foundation choice goes as follows: MATCH THE YELLOW-BROWN UNDERTONE OF THE SKIN EXACTLY, EXCEPT WHEN:

1. THE FACE IS LIGHTER THAN THE NECK. THEN IT WILL BE NECESSARY TO CHOOSE A FOUNDATION THAT IS DARKER THAN THE FACE.

2. WHEN THE FACE IS DARKER THAN THE NECK. THEN YOU WILL NEED TO USE A FOUNDATION TO LIGHTEN THE FACE. ALWAYS AVOID AREAS OF DEMARCATION BETWEEN THE NECK AND THE FACE.

Types of Foundation

There are four types of foundation: oil-free, water-based, oil-based, and grease-stick. Pancake (an oil-free type of foundation) and grease-stick are for theatrical purposes. Pancake works with water. It is applied while wet and then dries quickly. Grease-stick is heavy and thick in texture, like a cover stick applied to the entire face. These are not typically used by most women, so the focus will be on the other three types of foundation.

Oil-Free

Oil-free makeup has no oil in it whatsoever and can take two forms: One is watery and contains mostly talc, water, alcohol and coloring. The other looks like a traditional, creamy, thick foundation which contains water, propylene glycol (a slip agent) and waxes.

Oil-free makeup that is creamy in texture rather than watery, goes on heavy and wet, drying into place with a solid finish that shows no reflection or shine. This is a good choice for photography and television where you do not want to shine. It will also last much longer on oily skin than any other foundation type which, for some women, is very desirable.

The disadvantage of the creamy oil-free foundation is that it goes on so heavy and dry and it creates a mask-like appearance and feeling on the face. This is very, very heavy makeup. This is the type of foundation I wear for television appearances, so from personal experience, I know that while applying, you must blend quickly as it dries in place very fast. Once it's blended on it won't move; you have to get it right the first time. Adding water to your sponge to make this foundation go on thinner tends to make oil-free foundation streak. In terms of applying shadow and blush, this foundation is also more difficult to work over. Because oil-free makeup has no movement (oil in a foundation allows for movement) the powder will stick to the surface which makes blending difficult and correcting mistakes a nightmare.

Oil-free makeups that contain alcohol should not be used. The alcohol content irritates the skin, which increases oil production and dries out the skin at the same time; the very things you were hoping to avoid. They also go on very thinly and watery. After applying, when the water and alcohol evaporate leaving the colored talc behind, the talc adheres to the skin poorly and the desired goal for even coverage is no longer possible.

Water-Based

Water-based does *not* mean oil-free; it simply means that the first ingredient is water, and the second or third is usually oil. (Oil-based is the reverse: The first ingredient is oil and the second, usually, is water.)

A water-based foundation is a lightweight product. You don't need to add water when applying because it is already the right consistency. It can go on in a beautiful, even, thin layer. (If you want heavy coverage you will probably be disappointed in a water-based foundation.) Water-based foundation is the perfect type to wear alone without the aid of a moisturizer. As I mentioned earlier, when the foundation and moisturizer contain many of the same ingredients, there is no need to wear both and water-based foundations usually fit the bill.

I personally don't feel there are any major disadvantages to water-based foundations and I recommend them wholeheartedly. A consumer perceived disadvantage is that it contains oil, and women with oily skin will show shine quickly. Most women have a media-induced hate of shine from oil in any amount. (It seems shininess is horrible unless, of course, it is in the form of shiny eyeshadows, shiny blushes and not the nose or face.) Yet, if you still have issues over shine, and that's truly understandable, then a loose powder can be worn all over the face to reduce the glow.

Oil-Based

Oil-based foundation has many of the same properties as water-based foundation, except that the first two ingredients are reversed, oil comes first and water is second or third. Oil-based tends to be heavier, thicker, and greasier than water-based. It can be great for women with very dry skin who also want more coverage from their makeup. Be careful with wearing powder over this type of foundation. The oil will grab the talc and the face can appear thick and heavily madeup. The typical recommendation with these products is to add water to your sponge so that it goes on thinner which means it will be more like water-based foundations. Why not use that in the first place?

NOTE: *For women of color, including those with dark tans, oil-based foundation may make you look greasy or orange. With too flat a foundation, one that has no oil, you can look grey and ashy. If you're one of these women, water-based foundation may be the best option.*

Which One Is For You?

If what you want from a foundation is one that goes on easily, looks smooth and even, shows as few flaws as possible, gives the rest of the makeup something to adhere to without looking as though you're wearing a mask, then (if you haven't guessed by now) you should choose a water-based foundation. The pros definitely outweigh any negatives. The exception is when skin is very oily. Then the creamy type of oil-free foundation is good to use. Not wonderful, but better than water-based.

Shopping for foundation can be very tricky and I am totally sympathetic because I know how difficult this can be. There is truly only one way to prevent buying the wrong color: Try it before you buy it. Do that by shopping for makeup without makeup on, or at least be willing to remove it when you get to the cosmetic counter. It does no good to put makeup on over your other makeup. All that tells you is how the makeup will look when worn over other makeup. Also, do not try foundation or any other cosmetic for that matter, on your arm, wrist, or any other part of your anatomy besides your face. Your arm is not your face. You're trying to match the color to your face and neck which is a completely different tone than your hand or arm.

Consider it this way; you wouldn't shop for a new item of clothing by putting it on over the clothing you already had on, would you? And you wouldn't try a blouse on over your left leg to see if it fits! The same is true for your face. You must experiment with makeup types and color on a clean face to really see the effect of the cosmetics you might be buying.

Powdering

Powdering the face after foundation is applied is optional, though not necessary. I personally like some amount of glow on the skin. To me, that represents healthy, glowing, alive, young skin. Skin that shows no signs of reflection looks dull and dry. I know there are levels between looking dry and looking like a jar of chicken fat (kind of like you can see your own reflection on your face). But if you avoid a moisturizer and blend your foundation smoothly with a sponge, the amount of shine should be just perfect. I encourage you to try not powdering when makeup is fresh at the beginning of the day. Rather, use it after the day goes by when touching up makeup. As your own natural oil spreads over the face during the day, powder will help reduce that oily intensity.

When powdering use a large, full, round brush. Pick up some of the powder on the full of the brush and apply in the same motion and direction you did the foundation. That will keep everything going in the same direction and retain an even appearance. Before powdering you can use your sponge or a tissue to dab off excess oil from the face.

I strongly recommend translucent powder as opposed to any of the pressed powders or talcs presently on the market for this purpose. Pressed powders contain wax (that's what they're pressed with), and you don't need to dust the face with both the powder and wax.

Brushes

All cosmetics have an appropriate tool that is essential to the application of that particular product. One of the major tools is the brush. Not those little doll-sized applicators or sponge-tip sticks that come with cosmetics, but good, full-sized, thick haired, soft bristle brushes to help assure good even application of the contour, blush and eye makeup. This is as good a time as any to throw away those little brushes that come in blush compacts that are too small to match the size of anyone's cheek.

c) **Proper Use of Brushes**

Eyeliner

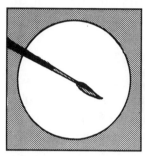

DO
Use the flat
side of the
brush.

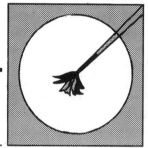

DO NOT
Use the tip.
Do not
splay the
brush.

Eyeshadow

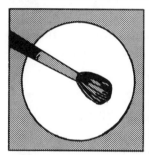

DO
Use the flat
edge of the
brush.

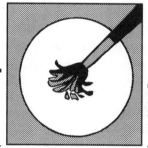

DO NOT
Splay the
brush.

Blush, Powder or Contour

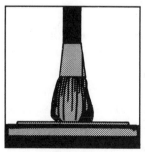

DO
Use the full
head of the
brush.

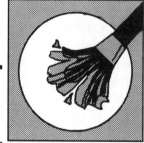

DO NOT
Splay the
brush.

The rule for choosing the right brush is: *The brush should match the job and size of the area it is to be used on!* A wise investment in any makeup case would be good brushes. Brushes should not be so stiff they scratch the face and yet not so soft as to be difficult to control. A good brush can make all the difference between a quick, smooth makeup job and a sloppy, time-consuming makeup application.

Whenever you can see a line where the brush stroke was placed, or feel an urge to use your hand to blend what you've just applied, you are most likely not using the brush properly or your brush is too stiff for soft application and blending. (You may also have applied your foundation poorly which means you need to read over the section on sponges again.) You should not be blending anything with your fingers; only your brush or the flat, square, thin sponge you used to apply your foundation. Blending is the key to good looking makeup. That requires not only good brushes but good techniques; not the wild beating a lot of women struggle with when they put on their blush and eyeshadows.

The tendency is to use the brush in a rubbing or wiping motion on the face. There truly is an easier way. Here are two reliable techniques to follow: *Do not wipe or beat the brush against the face.* Inadvertently you may be wiping off what you just put on, not to mention the foundation underneath. *Do brush in short, quick motions gliding over the skin.*

Something else that is critical to good application, even though it may seem insignificant at first, is the way you pick up the powder on your brush before you apply it. Never smash your brush into the powder. Rather place your brush into the powder gently, without moving the bristles. You don't want to see the brush hair splay. (See diagram C) Always stroke through the powder evenly and be sure to always knock the excess powder off before you apply it to the face. Knocking the excess off prevents applying too much color to the first place your brush touches on the face.

Contouring

Contouring was very popular during the middle and late 70s. If you didn't have sunken hollows just above the jaw and right below the cheekbone or didn't know how to create that look, you were doomed to exist with a round, full, unfashionable face. I remember those days vividly; everyone searching in vain for their cheekbone. Thank goodness the popularity of contouring to reshape the face has since died down. A probable reason for its demise is that believable-looking contouring is a difficult part of makeup application. It takes a certain amount of skill and patience, which is more than most women have time to deal with every morning before starting their day or going to work. What often happens is cheek contour ends up looking like a stripe of brown powder under a stripe of blush. Before making this step a part of your daily routine, practice, practice, practice.

If you choose to contour, it is always a separate step and color from blush application. Pinks, reds, and oranges are used in blushing. Only brown tones are used in contouring. Choosing whether you use a red-brown, yellow-brown, or a grey-brown depends on the other colors of lipstick, blush and eyeshadow you will be wearing. (How to choose color will be discussed thoroughly later.)

The traditional areas you can choose to contour are under the cheekbone, at the sides of the forehead (temple area) and down the sides of the nose. There are some rules of placement to help you find and apply the areas to be contoured.

NOTE: *I am not going to recommend contouring or shading along any portion of the jawline.* After going through all the trouble to find a foundation that leaves no line of demarcation at the jaw, it makes no sense to draw a brown stripe there and hope people believe it looks like natural shadow. Plus, the likelihood that makeup in this area will end up on your collar is about 100%.

Under the Cheekbone

To find this area, start your contouring shade no further in than the pupil, and no further down than the area just above the corner of the mouth. At that intersection, about a quarter-inch behind the laugh line, place your brush and stroke the color straight back towards the middle of the ear. You will find that this is just under the cheekbone. (See diagram D) This area is approximately one-half inch in width, yet there should be no definite edges visible. Use your sponge to soften hard edges.

The starting point for under-cheekbone contouring is almost always the same, but your end point at the ear can vary depending on the effect you desire. The steeper the angle of contour going towards the top of the ear, the longer the face will appear. A square or round face might want to experiment contouring with a steeper angle. The longer the face, as an

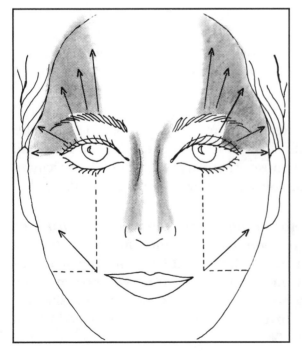

D) CONTOURING
Soften hard edges with your sponge. For temple contour reapply if needed to soften eyeshadow. Under cheekbone and nose, contouring is optional.

oblong or triangular face tends to be, the more straight back towards the middle of the ear the line can be, to de-emphasize the length by bisecting the face.

CAUTION: BE SURE TO NEVER DROP THE CONTOUR COLOR BELOW THE MOUTH OR RAISE IT ONTO THE CHEEK-BONE ITSELF. By the way, the technique of sucking in the sides of your mouth to help find your cheekbone will only help to find the sides of your mouth, not your cheekbone.

Recommendation: The contour brush I recommend is the brush usually labeled for blush or rouge. The blush brush is too small for most cheeks and the contour brush is too hard and flat for contour, which makes hard, visible edges. Using the full of the rouge brush, knocking off the excess powder before applying and brushing in short quick motions going back to the ear, should net the best results.

Sides of the Nose

The trick here is to be sure not to blend the color out into the area under the eyes or on the face. Keep the color restricted to the sides of the nose. A good technique to assist you while practicing is to place your index finger flat down the center of the nose, then lay your brush along the side of it. Where the brush falls against your finger is the area to be contoured. Softly apply this color fully around the tip of the nose, on the flare of the nostrils and continue it up under the eyebrow avoiding the tear drop area. (See diagram D) This end point under the eyebrow will be an overlap area when you start applying your eyeshadows. For the nose contour, either use a large flat eyeshadow brush or use the brush you used for the under-cheek-bone contour and pinch it thin enough to accommodate the sides of the nose.

Contouring the nose has nothing to do with whether the nose is large or small. There's a much more artistic reason for using this shading technique. If you're applying a full, classic makeup, and you ignore the nose, you will have color everywhere and a white blotch in the center of the face. Con-touring the nose helps to achieve color balance for the rest of the face.

Temple Contour

This is a very traditional step in makeup. As essential as mascara and as basic as blush. In any fashion magazine you will notice the models have this step applied. This step shades the back of the under eyebrow bone, out and up onto the forehead, like a pie wedge without the edges. The color is applied under the back third of the eyebrow and then brushed all the way back to the hairline about three inches wide at its fullest point. (See diagram D) This technique creates an area of color to blend eyeshadow into. With temple contour neatly applied, the eyeshadow at the back of the eye doesn't abruptly end as a harsh colored edge in mid, flesh-colored, temple. Without temple contour the forehead becomes a great white wall against the color background of the cheeks and eyes.

CAUTION: The things that make temple shading go wrong is forgetting that this step overlaps the back third under eyebrow, brushes over the eyebrow itself and then goes strtaight back to the hair and then up onto the forehead in a three inch spread. This is a shaded area like the blush and it should never look like a stripe.

Blushing

Blushing is such an important obvious part of the makeup that to see it painted on like highway dividers is very frustrating. I urge you to take your time with this step. When this is on wrong, no one notices anything else.

The parameters for finding the areas to be blushed are almost the same as for contouring under the cheekbone. Using this method is a fail-safe way to apply blush. Start your brush at the intersection of the pupil and the tip of the nose. This will be approximately a quarter to a half-inch behind the laugh line. Place the full of the brush here and then, brush DOWN-WARDS and back towards the center of your ear, applying the color gently as you go. (See diagram E) Brushing down as opposed to back and forth will eliminate achieving a stripe effect instead of a blush effect. And as always you have your handy dandy little sponge nearby to soften edges.

Blush safety check: Brush usage is downward rather than straight back, covering an area that is approximately one and a half inches wide. Never blush the lines around the eye as it makes them look more evident, as well as red and irritated. It isn't necessary to blush around the eye area at all. Also do not blush below the mouth, that's too much color and be sure to avoid blushing the laugh lines and making them look more obvious. If you are applying both blush and under-cheekbone contour you can apply the contour color first and then blend the blush on top of and gradually down, into the contour color. Then, using your sponge, you blend until you creatively meld the colors together into an attractive design. (An attractive design means not being able to tell where one color stops and the other color starts.)

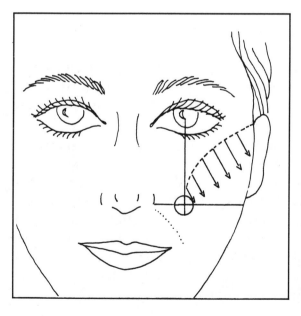

E) BLUSH PLACEMENT
Brush down and proceed back to ear. Do not blush by laugh lines or below mouth.

Blush is for the cheekbone. You never blush your nose, forehead, hairline or chin. Red noses are something you have after a cold, not something you apply to your face. Please avoid stripes of blush down the center of the forehead and chin as well. It's like wearing a shoe on your hand — that just isn't where it was intended to go. And whose hairline is really ever pink?

Lipstick and Lipliner

When you use lipstick or lip liner, always follow the actual outline of your lips and mouth. Please do not use corrective techniques to make the mouth look larger or longer, especially for daytime makeup. These techniques are not only difficult, but if you try to change the outline of your mouth and make it look fuller, an hour or two later your lipstick will wear off and your lip liner will look like you missed your mouth. It really can look like you got up late and just missed your lips. Always line the lips using the actual shape, then fill in with your lipstick color.

FASHION NOTE: *Lip liner stopped being an obvious, dark, brown, definite line around the mouth in 1978. Lip liner for a contemporary fashion look should not show obviously at all.* Brown lipstick is also, thank heaven, out of date. Brown lip liners and lipstick weren't an attractive color when they were in fashion. Browns and cranberries, especially on thin lips, make the lips look severe and harsh, like Dracula lips. Warm or cool bright colors may take a bit to get used to, but once you do, they truly make a mouth look softer and more attractive.

Try to avoid greasy lipsticks and lip glosses if you have a problem with your lipstick bleeding. The greasier the lipstick, gloss and/or lip liner, the faster it will run and bleed into the lines around the mouth. Drier feeling lipsticks are best for conquering this problem. Powdering the mouth before the lipstick also helps. Another trick is to line the mouth slightly smaller than it actually is. This technique takes into account that lipstick moves as you wear it, so why start out placing the color where it will eventually end up anyway?

There is no truth to the rumor that using a lipstick brush helps keep the lipstick on longer. Putting on a lot of lipstick or wearing vivid strong colors and avoiding lip glosses keeps the lipstick on longer. (Another option is to try the new "prevent-lipstick-bleeding" products on the market. They don't work for everyone, but some women swear by them.)

Before I talk about choosing colors, it is important to explain some basic theories on just how to do that.

Fashion Makeup Means Choosing Colors that go Together

It is obvious from the sheer number of possible makeup looks in magazines today, that there is no one universally accepted opinion as to the proper way to combine color. In fact, there are so many differing options and preferences that it's not only unlikely to find the perfect combination, but unnecessary. Just as you don't wear the same colors of clothing everyday, the same is true for your makeup. Yet there are ways to go about making some good choices. Here are some of the most effective and aesthetically reliable options.

RULE NUMBER ONE: *Dress your face the same way you would dress your body.* If you wouldn't consider wearing a pink skirt with a blue blouse and an orange jacket, don't wear those colors on your face. This means avoid wearing orange lipstick, blue eyeshadow and pink blush. It even sounds distracting. Work monochromatically when using makeup colors for the lips, cheeks and eyes. Dress your face so it doesn't clash with itself. If your blush and eyeshadows are in the mauve/lavender family, so should the lip color be either pink or mauve or some shade of soft blue red. If your blush and eyeshadows are rust, brown and peach in color, so should the lipstick be either peach, rust, pale orange or red with yellow in it.

RULE NUMBER TWO: *Dress your face so it doesn't clash with what you wear.* Matching makeup to your clothing is important. (You wouldn't wear a pair of orange shoes with a pink outfit.) What you're looking to match is the undertone of of your clothing; blue or pink tones vs. yellow or green tones. Blue tones mean shades of purple, mauve, pink, lavender, and the like. Yellow tones mean peach, coral, orange, rust and the like. When wearing a particular color of clothing your makeup should coordinate with that particular color family.

Now that doesn't mean blue skirt, blue eyeshadow any more than it means to wear a blue lipstick. Besides that rule about blue outfit, blue eyeshadow falls apart when you wear a black, navy or red and white striped outfit. Choosing blue tones in makeup colors means using shades of lipstick, blush or eyeshadow color that are blue-toned (not blue) and for yellow tones that means using makeup colors that are yellow-toned (not yellow). *All colors, depending on how much blue or yellow they contain, can be either a yellow undertone or a blue undertone.* When grey is yellow-toned it appears drab or ashy-green. When grey is blue-toned it appears charcoal or slate-grey. When brown is blue-toned it may appear rosy-brown or mauve-brown. When brown is yellow-toned it can appear neutral-beige to golden tan.

When your wardrobe is mostly neutral, without being over-whelmingly blue or yellow-toned, you have a lot less to worry about when choosing makeup colors. Clothing will clash with your makeup if it is an obvious color mismatch like pink blouse, orange lipstick or peach blouse, rose blush. Even though grays, blacks, tans and neutral colors of clothing do indeed have blue and yellow undertones, because they tend to be less obvious, they rarely clash with any color of makeup.

RULE NUMBER THREE: *Do not wear colors that are more intense or less intense than you are.* For those of you who haven't been "seasoned" yet, (discovered what clothing colors are best suited to your skin and hair color) or even if you have been, consider this simple, basic color compatibility theory: If you're a blonde with fair skin, cobalt blue or fushia will overwhelm you. If you are dark-haired and have dark skin, pale-blue or pink will make you look pale and blah. If you are blonde and have dark skin, vibrant but less intense colors would work and that would apply to dark-haired women with fair skin.

Red-heads or auburn-haired women almost always look better in vibrant colors that are yellow based. When considering color, focus as much on color choice as color intensity.

It is important to think of makeup as a fashion accessory and follow this rule of matching clothing color with makeup color. Even if the outfit you wear is a color that is not the most flattering for you, it is still necessary to find makeup colors that will not clash. For example, if you wear a vibrant purple outfit and your better color is lavender, choose eyeshadows that are lavender-grey in appearance or a pale pink blush that has more ash tones than vibrant pink and do the same for the lipstick. Those makeup colors will work with your outfit, and be soft enough to go with your skin tone. The same would be true for a woman who is wearing brown earth tones but should be wearing more vibrant colors like purple. In this situation choose colors of blush and lipstick that are more coral or peachy-pink, and shadows that have more charcoal-grey than brown which would still work with both the outfit and your skin tone.

The Agony and the Ecstasy — Choosing Color

Choosing color can have its agonies even when you know all the rules. You need not only be cautious of how your makeup and clothing coordinate, you also need to be aware that makeup is not static on the skin. Skin color so blatantly affects the makeup colors you wear that you need to take that into consideration along with what clothing colors you will be wearing.

On skin that has high yellow-brown tones or ashy green tones, always avoid reinforcing those tones by using shades of orange, yellow or grey-green in the makeup (rusts, ochre, etc.). Same goes for skin with intense redness. Why put on more red with shades of pink or rose blush and lipstick and make the skin look redder?

A person with ruddy skin color that needs to match a blue-toned outfit can choose makeup colors that are muted shades of grey, grey-brown, mauve-brown and grey-lavender tones to soften the redness.

A person with golden skin color (a much better word than sallow) that needs to match a yellow undertoned outfit can choose makeup colors that are bright peachy-pink and coral that won't dull the skin.

Olive skin color can follow the same suggestions for golden skin color. (But it's really best to never wear anything that has any yellow tones or dull muted shades to it at all.)

Is Fashion Awareness for Everyone?

I get a lot of people who, at this point say to me, "I don't want things that are fashionable. I just want to look good." Sorry, it's hard to have one without the other. For example, you might have looked really good in go-go boots and Nehru jackets twenty odd years ago, but today, chances are you are going to look out of place. Why? Because they are out of date and no longer fashionable to wear. What is fashionable today is directly related to what looks good. Yet, within any fashion statement there are lots of clothing options to choose from that will look great on you.

The same follows for makeup. Remember wearing "Twiggy" lashes drawn on under your lower lashes? False eyelashes, or thin plastic liner on the eyelid? Or maybe you recall when white under the eyebrow, dark brown in the creases and white or blue on the eyelid was all the rage? (It was and still is very hard to blend very different colors together. As a result those colors always looked like stripes of white, brown and blue stuck on the face in an obvious manner. Not only that, but white under the brow makes that area look puffy and saggy and who needs a puffy, saggy brow bone?)

Of course, nowadays the problem isn't so much trying to avoid wearing "Twiggy" lashes or blue, brown and white shadow combinations. Cosmetic companies haven't sold those colors together for awhile. Rather it's the trio of colors like bright yellow and green or rose pink and blue that they try to sell that need to be avoided.

Blue Eyeshadow Should be *Illegal*

This is the perfect time to mention why, in my opinion, bright blue eyeshadow should be illegal. (Now where have you heard that before?) Blue is probably the most misused color women wear on their faces, although shiny lime green shadows and bright shiny pink run a close second with rosy, orange foundation not far behind. But blue wins hands down because it is sold more than any other color in the country. (Do you get the feeling I might be fighting a losing battle?)

Solid blue splashed across the lid or worse, painted all over the eye from the lashes to the brow, flashes out from the eye area like a neon sign. Blue has a hard time blending with any other color so it always tends to stand out and becomes more obvious than anything else you may have on. Think about it for a second; walking down the aisle of a local grocery store or department store you see a woman walking toward you with a stripe of blue across her lid. Think about how that looks. You can see that blue stripe a mile away! Not her eyes, not her face, just her blue eyeshadow.

In all fairness, I'm referring mostly to a complete solid covering of the eyelid with blue shadow or a bright blue eyeliner, thickly wrapped around the lashes. A little shading at the back of the eye, or a little lining with navy or grey-blue, if done properly and with restraint, isn't the worst thing I can think of. (See, I really *can* be flexible.) If you feel you get compliments on your blue eyeshadow or liner then definitely you're doing something wrong. You want people to compliment you, not your makeup. Also take the time to flip through a fashion magazine and notice that none of the fashion layouts (the ads for the fashion designers, not the makeup ads) have models wearing blue eyeshadow, so why are you?

Eyeshadow Application

NOTE: *See large eye diagram for location of specific terms used in the eye design descriptions.*

Eyeshadow, as far as application technique goes, is applied almost completely opposite to the blush and contour. With eyeshadows, you use the flat of the brush, and apply with long,

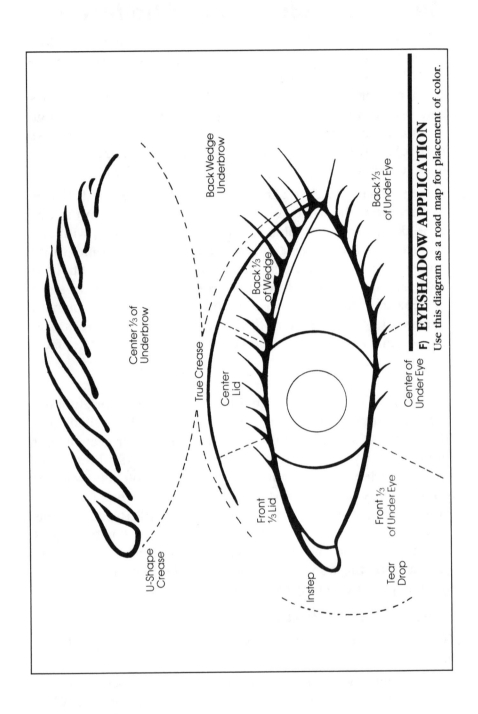

F) EYESHADOW APPLICATION

Use this diagram as a road map for placement of color.

Back Wedge Underbrow

Center 1/3 of Underbrow

True Crease

Center Lid

Front 1/3 Lid

U-Shape Crease

Back 1/3 of Wedge

Back 1/3 of Under Eye

Center of Under Eye

Front 1/3 of Under Eye

Instep

Tear Drop

stroking motions. In action, you are striping on the color, over-lapping each stroke until an even well blended appearance is achieved over the entire eye area. That means avoiding the use of brushes that have hard bristles or you will end up with hard lines. As always, the size of the brush matches the size of the area you're working on; the bigger the lid, the bigger the brush; the smaller the lid, the smaller the brush — and I mean brushes, not sponge tip applicators.

When trying to choose which eyeshadow color and tone goes where, there are two general rules to always keep in mind that can get you started in the right direction: THE BIGGER THE EYELID, THE DARKER OR DEEPER THE COLOR CAN BE. THE SMALLER THE EYELID, THE BRIGHTER OR MORE COL-ORFUL TONES CAN BE USED. (Never use shiny white.) This is a totally logical approach. If the eyelid is already prominent it isn't necessary to make it appear any bigger (it's kind of like a busty woman wearing falsies, it's overdoing what's already overdone), and if the eyelid is small it is more than appropriate to put on a color that stands out more.

The same rule applies for under the eyebrow. THE SMAL-LER THE UNDER-EYEBROW AREA, THE BRIGHTER THE COLOR SHOULD BE. THE LARGER THE AREA BETWEEN THE EYEBROW AND THE CREASE, THE DEEPER OR DARKER THE COLOR SHOULD BE. (Always avoid wearing white.) You guess-ed it, the busty woman analogy applies here as well.

REMINDER: Be cautious of "rules" that are formulated as a way to correct problems like eyes being too close together or too far apart. Who said close-set eyes are any better than eyes set further apart.

The two major areas where eyeshadow is always applied, regardless of design, are the lid and under-eyebrow. The lid is fairly obvious, you only need to be sure that there are no patches of skin showing through at the inside corner of the eye next to the lashes and do not extend the color into the tear drop or out beyond the lashes.

The under-eyebrow is a little more complicated. This area starts at the instep of the eye, where the eyebrow begins, next to the bridge of the nose. If you were doing a nose contour, that's where the contour would stop and the eyeshadow would start. Regardless of whether you're contouring the nose or not, the underbrow color starts there anyway. (With the nose right there it provides a natural indentation that hides the beginning edge of your eyeshadow.) The eyeshadow moves from that inner corner by the nose, down to the crease, blending out and across to the end of the brow and out into the temple contour. (See diagram F) That's what the temple contour is there for, so we don't see where your eye makeup starts and stops. (The placement and blending for other design options will be explained later.)

Designing the Eye

There are dozens of eye designs from which to choose that will create all kinds of effects. Yet almost all designs, from one extent to another, use any combination of the following basic designs as a way to shape their drama; a one-color, two-color, three-color, four-color or five-color eye design. For a classic design you would apply each additional color in order, completing up to and including the five-color eye design.

Your own ability, personal preference and time consideration is the basis for choosing which eye design to start with. For example, if you're new to makeup, or prefer a near no-makeup look, use the one-color design with an eyeliner and temple contour. If you're used to wearing makeup, try the four or five-color design.

The designs listed are a step-by-step building block for completing a formal eye design. Yet, each by itself is a full design when worn with eyeliner, temple contour and mascara.

One-Color Eye Design

One color is applied all over the eye area from the lashes to the under-eyebrow. Liner and temple contour are required to complete the design. This single color should be a soft tan or neutral taupe, something definitely not obvious. Always avoid carrying a bright color all over the eye.

Two-Color Eye Design

One-color is applied fully on the eyelid, and another color is applied fully from the crease to the brow. (The lid color and under-eyebrow color meet in the crease.) A liner and temple contour are required to complete the design. To decide where to put your color choices use the rule for color placement intensity on page 71.

Three-Color Eye Design

Start with the two-color eye design and add either a back-wedge or U-shaped crease design. (See explanation on page 75.) The lid and under-eyebrow color are softer and less intense than the wedge or U-shaped crease color. A full design would include a temple contour and eyeliner. (See diagram I)

Four-Color Eye Design

Start with the two-color eye design, then add a U-shaped crease color and a back-wedge. When both a U-shaped crease color and a back-wedge are used, the back-wedge color is more intense or darker than the crease color.

NOTE: *Notice on the diagram that this U-shaped crease color always includes a back-wedge design so the shading doesn't look like a wing hanging out in mid-air.* The difference then between a four-color eye design and a three-color eye design is the former uses an extra and darker back-wedge color that is different from the U-shaped crease design to build depth and interest. When executing the three-color design, you use either a back-wedge alone or a U-shaped crease color and back-wedge that are the same color.

Five-Color Eye Design

Start with a two-color eye design, add a back-wedge color, a U-shaped crease color and last, a true crease color (see explanation on page 76) in order of least intense color to most intense color; the lid and under-eyebrow are light, the U-shaped crease color is next softest and the wedge and true crease are the most intense.

Back-Wedge and Full Back-Wedge

This is an accent color which shades the back ⅓ corner of the lid. A full back-wedge shades the back ⅓ corner of the lid, blending softly into the crease and out towards the back ⅓ of the under-eyebrow.

The trick to getting this design on correctly is to be sure that the most intense placement of color is on the back ⅓ of the lid. (See diagrams below) The softest part of the color placement is the area nearest the eyebrow.

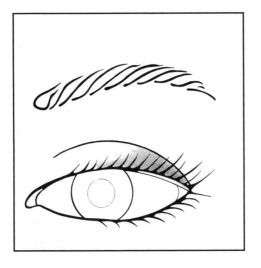

G) WEDGE
Shade the back ⅓ of the lid only.

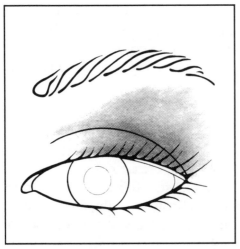

H) FULL BACK WEDGE
Shade from back ⅓ of lid out to the back ⅓ of the under eyebrow. Temple contour blends out back edge of eyeshadow.

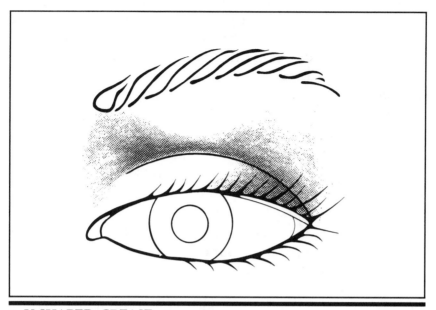

I) U-SHAPED CREASE
This design always includes a Full Back Wedge

The trick to getting this design on correctly is to be sure that the most intense placement of color is on the back ⅓ of the lid. (See diagram H) The softest part of the color placement is the area nearest the eyebrow.

The more dramatic the design, the more dramatic the color that can be used and/or the further away from the crease toward the back ⅓ of the under-eyebrow it can be blended. Another hint to doing this correctly is to watch the angle away from the lid, toward the under-eyebrow, as you do your blending. The softer the angle up, the softer the appearance. The more severe the angle, either straight up or straight out, the harder or more dramatic the effect.

U-Shaped Crease

The U-shaped crease design is a wonderful design, but very difficult to accomplish. Part of the difficulty is because the shadow travels across the entire eye from the front ⅓ of the under-eyebrow dropping abruptly down to the center true crease area, then gradually blends back up again to the back ⅓ of the under-eyebrow and then blends out into the temple contour. It is this dip in the center that makes this design difficult, as does deciding when to start the movement back up from the center toward the eyebrow. (See diagram I) Be careful to keep the area under the front ⅓ of the under-eyebrow soft and well blended.

I vacillate between calling this design a "U-shape" or an "S-shape" design. When you look at the finished design it resembles a "U", but when applying, it goes on like an "S" due to the curved shaped front ⅓ of the under-eyebrow where the design starts.

Suggestions for good application are: The center crease area is the darkest, so start your brush there and blend out and up to the front or back ⅓ of the under-eyebrow from this point. The softest part of this design is the front and back ⅓ of the under-eyebrow, so be careful not to build too much color in those areas.

The way to decide when to start blending the center crease up toward the front and back ⅓ of the underbrow is when the crease starts curving down. Wait, that's not quite as confusing as it sounds. Look at your eye in a mirror. Now find your crease. Notice the center is the highest point and the sides curve down from there. Where the curve down starts from this high center point you begin your blending (movement with the brush) up toward the back ⅓ of the under-eyebrow or up toward the front ⅓ of the under-eyebrow. That gives the illusion of lifting and opening the eye.

True Crease

A five-color eye design adds a true crease color to the full four-color eye design application. It is a deep color used in the fold of the eye that then connects with the back-wedge on the lid. (See diagram F) The true crease color is placed below the U-shaped crease color and is a more intense color than the U-shaped crease color. When the back-wedge color is different (and, of course darker than the U-shaped crease color) the true crease color can be the same as the back-wedge.

REMEMBER: Watch your blending. You're actually never as concerned with where your makeup starts and stops as you are with how each application of shadow overlaps and blends into the other. What you want is smooth movement, so that the eye travels over the face without stopping or tripping over lines, stripes, patches or streaks.

WARNING: TO MAKE THIS WHOLE PROCESS AS EASY AS POSSIBLE, USE COLORS THAT ARE EASY TO BLEND (explanation on page 87). Always use the temple contour brush and not your sponge to soften the back edge of your eye makeup, and avoid like the plague glittery, irridescent, shiny, sparkly eyeshadows. Glittery eyeshadows exaggerate the lines in the eye area and make you look wrinkly even if you don't have wrinkles.

Eyeliners

From 1969 to 1974 we progressed from wearing liquid liner with wings to wearing "Twiggy" lashes without lines for a fashionable look. Then somewhere around 1976, the smudge pencils came into fashion. The smudge stick was great. It was fast and convenient. Unfortunately, it was also impossible to sharpen and it did just what it said it was going to do; it smudged all over the place. Smeared eye makeup was a definite problem.

Then there was the period where a fashionable eye was one where the liner was placed on the rim, inside the eye. We were told that placing the pencil here would make the white of the eye appear whiter. Nothing could be further from the truth. With constant application of a foreign substance in the eye, the resulting irritation leaves the eye bloodshot. Plus this lovely effect of lining the inside rim only lasts about one hour and then the color clumps up at the inside corner of the eye and smears under the eye. Clumpy, smeary and bloodshot eyes are never fashionable or attractive. Thank goodness during the '80s the fashion became a more specific line around the outside of the eyes, and that's pretty much where we are today in respect to eye lining.

Because of all the problems I mentioned earlier with regard to pencils, I never use pencils when lining the eye. It is very hard to control the size of the line with a fat-tipped pencil or even a thin-tipped pencil that refuses to sharpen. But not so with a brush. So whenever you're lining the eyes I strongly recommend using a deep, vivid colored eyeshadow powder and a tiny brush. Another benefit of using powder and a brush is that you can always use the powder as an eyeshadow or contour, depending on the color, by just changing the brush size.

Always line the eyes last, after the eyeshadow is applied. Use a thin, slightly stiff brush. Whether you use your powder wet or dry (preferably dry), stroke the brush through the color, keeping the bristles together. Don't dab or rub the brush into the color. Move it across the shadow in the direction of the bristles, making sure the form of the brush is not destroyed. (See diagram C, page 57) Be patient, this technique takes longer than a pencil.

When lining the eyelid, make the line a solid, even line going thin at the front ⅓ of the lid to thicker at the back ⅓ of the lid if you wish. You can line all the way across the eye from the inside corner to the outer edge, or you can choose to stop the line where the lashes stop and start. (I prefer to line all the way across.)

Along the lower lashes, I line only the outer ⅔ with a softer color than the liner used on the lid. I rarely close up the inside corner of the eye by lining all the way around in a complete circle. That could be a more dramatic look or a good technique for large eyes. Lining all the way underneath the eye tends to create an eyeglass look around the eye, and strongly changes the definition and softness. It can make the eyeliner the stronger statement rather than the eye itself.

The general rule for choosing eyeliner color is to choose a brown, grey or black shade. Eyeliner is meant to give depth to lashes and to make them appear thicker. If the liner is a bright or true pastel color, the attention will be focused past the lashes to the color applied as opposed to the more defined, subtle, even flow from lashes to liner. Test it on yourself. Line one eye with a vibrant color, the other eye with a brown or black and see which one looks like it has thicker lashes. (Color liner can be used, but generally only under the lower lashes, and then I would still line with a dark brown or black at the base of the lashes. This is a two-layer eye lining technique and works well to create definition, and color intensity.)

The thickness and intensity of the liner on the lid depends on the size of the lid — the larger the lid, the thicker and softer the eyeliner should be. The smaller the lid, the thinner and more intense the liner should be. When your lid doesn't show, forget lining altogether.

Another important tip for getting eyeliner on correctly is to make sure the lower liner is less intense than the upper liner and that the two lines meet at the back corner of the eye. Do not extend the lines beyond the eye. Please, no eyeliner wings.

Mascara

Mascara is a wonderful invention and is considered basic to all makeup application. Many experts say that if you're not wearing any other makeup, at least wear mascara. Unfortunately, many of us (I'm guilty of this one too) get carried away and wear way too much mascara. (Women who have long lashes: Remember the "busty woman" analogy.)

The need to overdo lashes is probably because most women feel long lashes are to be coveted, and the cosmetic industry advertises this point to death on TV, in magazines and on labels and packaging. Yet, the more you apply doesn't mean the more beautiful you are. Actually, the more you apply, the greater the chance of mascara flaking or chipping and for the lashes to appear hard and spiked. The lashes can only take so much weight, and the excess weight can break them. Gunked up lashes with tons of mascara do not resemble long, thick lashes; they resemble gunked up mascara. Barred windows curled over the eye don't quite look like luscious lashes.

That brings up curling the lashes. The eyelash curler — a strange looking device I've never understood, not only places the lashes at a strange angle for the sake of making them look longer, it can end up breaking them and pulling them out. Doesn't that defeat the purpose of making your lashes look longer?

Mascara comes in three basic types: waterproof, water soluble, and lash-lengthening. I prefer water soluble only.

To remove waterproof mascara, you must pull and wipe at the eye because it is difficult to remove. Water soluble mascaras on the other hand, are easy to remove. They come off with just water and your cleanser with no need to pull or sag the skin. And when mascara falls into the eye, you really do want it to dissolve with water and not remain in its solid form to keep it from scratching the eye. Due to a lot of scratched corneas, it is hard to find mascaras that contain fibers anymore. Most lash-lengthening type mascaras nowadays are not all that different from any other mascara.

I apply mascara to the lower lashes by holding the wand perpendicular to the eye and parallel to the lashes, which avoids getting mascara on the cheek. This makes it easier to reach the lashes at both ends of the eye. Both the traditional application of mascara (round brushing the upper lashes from the base of the lash up) and holding the wand perpendicular at the edges can get all the lashes on the lid. An old, cleaned-up mascara wand can be used to separate lashes and remove clumps.

Mascara mistakes landing on the skin (which seems to be a daily inevitable occurance) can often be taken care of simply when you use water soluble mascara. Wait until the mistake dries completely, and then chip the mascara away with a cotton swab. Most of it will just flake off, with very little repair work needed. Always check for mascara smudges. They can look very sloppy and distracting.

The tendency for the mascara tube to dry up can be alleviated by not over-pumping the wand into the tube hoping to build up mascara on the brush. All that really accomplishes is pumping air into the tube which makes the product dry up faster. Another solution is to avoid the wide bristled brushes. In order to accommodate the wider brush, the tube opening needs to be larger, which will allow more air to get inside, which causes the mascara to dry out faster. (Don't be fooled by the hope that wider bristles will make lashes any longer. Usually the applicator is so big it's clumsy to use and harder to get the lashes at the corners.)

You can increase the life of your mascara by adding a drop of distilled water to the tube. This can be repeated several times until all the mascara is gone. (This, of course, applies only to water soluble mascara.)

Blue Lashes?

I'm not fond of blue, purple or green mascara. Aside from the fact that no one really has purple or blue lashes, this book isn't dealing with trendy makeup looks and purple lashes would hardly create a classic look. Mascara is meant to enhance the eyes, not the lashes. Colored mascara, like colored eyeliner, becomes a distraction and makes you look at the lashes separately from the eye. If you want the lashes to appear thick and shape the eye, it is important that the mascara be a similar intensity and color as the eyeliner so that they flow one to the other without separation. With that information, the only decision left is when should you use black, dark brown or light brown? You determine that choice by the color intensity of the makeup. If you're wearing black liner and dramatic eye makeup then wear black mascara. A soft daytime makeup is perfect for brown liner and dark brown mascara.

NOTE: *If you have blonde hair, blonde lashes and blonde eyebrows, use light brown mascara and a soft brown liner. A blonde woman with very dark brows and dark lashes can use black or dark brown mascara depending on the intensity of the rest of the makeup.*

Eyebrows

Did I finally mention eyebrows? Well it's about time. No other aspect of makeup has gone through such dramatic fashion changes as eyebrow styles. We've gone from over-tweezed, pencil thin, tortured brows to over-drawn thick brows to a very soft, easy, pain-free looking brow. In general, nowadays the idea is to think of natural eyebrows (not neanderthal; natural). A full natural eyebrow is not only more attractive, but it is easier to keep up, too. Today's eyebrow fashion frees women from having to tweeze every day or having a 5:00 shadow growing under their brows. Of course, that doesn't mean you should

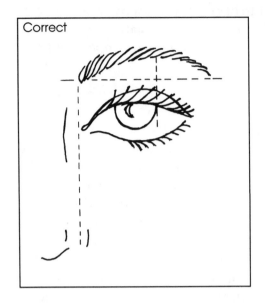

Correct

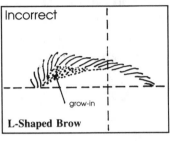

Incorrect

grow-in

L-Shaped Brow

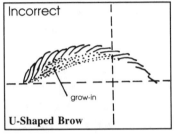

Incorrect

grow-in

U-Shaped Brow

J) EYEBROW

The eyebrow is correct when the arch falls over the back ⅓ of the eye and the front ⅓ of the brow starts from the center of the nostril.

L-Shaped Brow

Problem: Arch is over front ⅓ of brow.
   Cure: Grow in or powder indicated area.

U-Shaped Brow

Problem: No arch.
   Cure: Grow in or powder indicated area.

Over-Extended Brow (back)

Problem: Back ⅓ of brow is lower than front ⅓ of brow.
   Cure: Grow in or powder indicated area. Tweeze indicated area.

Over-Extended Brow (front)

Problem: Front ⅓ of brow is lower than back ⅓ of brow.
   Cure: Tweeze indicated area.

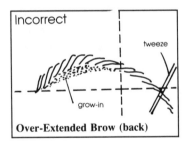

Incorrect

tweeze

grow-in

Over-Extended Brow (back)

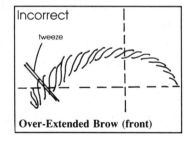

Incorrect

tweeze

Over-Extended Brow (front)

82

have one thick line of eyebrow growing across the bridge of the nose from one hairline to the other. There is a middle ground between Groucho Marx and Greta Garbo when it comes to the shape of your brows.

Discovering the shape of eyebrow that is best for you is very important because the shape and length of the eye itself is framed by the very appearance of the eyebrow. As much as a moustache can change the appearance of a man's face, so does the shape of an eyebrow affect a face. (Please no handle-bar eyebrows.)

The eyebrow gives the suggestion of the length and width of the eye. So, the further away from the nose you tweeze, the shorter the brow becomes and the smaller the eye appears. Your brow should begin along the center of the nostril. The arch should fall at the back ⅓ of the eye and although the eyebrow should be as long as possible, it still shouldn't go into the temple.The basic rule to follow is: THE FRONT PART OF THE BROW SHOULD NEVER DROP BELOW THE BACK PART OF THE BROW AND VICE VERSA! (See diagram J) Allowing this to happen, either with the way you tweeze your eyebrow or draw it on, makes you look like you're frowning or over-emphasizes the downward movement of the back part of the eye.

To apply eyebrow color, use a soft textured powder and a soft wedge brush. I never recommend using eyebrow pencils. They can produce a greasy look, tend to mat the hair, and usually look like a leftover from the 1930s. To apply the powder brow-color, brush the brow up with an old toothbrush and then apply the color with a wedge brush, first filling in the body of the brow, following the eyebrow hair exactly. A good rule to follow on where to place any extended color along the brow: If your eyebrows are set high, away from the eye, place the color under the eyebrow. The closer the brow is to the eye, the more you keep the color toward the top of the brow.

Shade no further than ¼ inch away from where the natural hair growth stops. No one believes that the line extended beyond the natural hair shape is brow. It simply looks very fake and accentuates the fact that there is no brow there in the first place.

Match the color you apply, to the brow color itself, rather than to hair color. You don't want to see a separation between the brow color and the shadow used to fill it in. If a woman has pale eyebrows and wants to darken the brow color, that's an option. But if she has red hair and brown eyebrows, using a red pencil or red color will look unnatural. A woman with blonde eyebrows may use a slightly darker blonde or ash-taupe color on her brows to make them visible. The goal is to use what we have as the basis for any makeup application, not to make an obvious theatrical change.

If you don't have a natural eyebrow to follow, use the wedge brush and powder and follow the bone above the eye, using what little hair there is. Usually there's enough shape to create a natural, shaded brow. Use a light touch, short quick motions, and avoid the temptation to exaggerate the shape, arch it severely, or extend it. Downplay the fact that there is no hair and don't over-exaggerate it with a strong, eye-catching line. Also, don't place a highlighter or light color under the brow to delineate further the placement of the brow color. Something dark next to something light makes it look more intense.

An option for sparse light-colored eyebrows is to brush mascara that matches the color of the brow, through the brow to make it appear thicker. It will take a few times to get the hang of it. You might have trouble at first controlling the amount fo mascara from the tube to the brow. Try using an old slightly dried up mascara instead of a new one. It will make it easier to apply the right amount. Give it a try; it really works.

Drippies

Last, but not least, after the eye design is completed, check for drippies under the eye and on the cheek with your sponge. Knocking off the excess from the brush every time helps prevent drippies but there's always one or two flakes that end up where they don't belong.

How Much Makeup?

It's completely up to you and the image you want to project. Makeup, like clothing, impacts the observer with a statement of intention. Wearing a business suit, instead of a jogging outfit to an office meeting makes a definite statement and it would make an even bigger statement if you were to do it the other way around. Because people react to the way we look and because makeup is a part of how we look, makeup, whether we like it or not, reveals something about who we are. So, to make sure it's saying what you want it to say, the concept of balance is essential to keep in mind when deciding what is right for you.

Balance refers back to the clothing confusion between wearing a business suit or jogging suit to the wrong occasion. Makeup coincides with those outfits the same way because it is a part of the outfit. Fully applied makeup with a jogging outfit is as inappropriate as no makeup with a business suit or an evening dress. Or look at it from this perspective; if you wouldn't wear a pair of high-heels with your jogging outfit, don't wear an evening type makeup with it either.

REMEMBER: When choosing makeup colors, the art of makeup is the flow of color and line on the face from one point to another so the viewer's eye never rests on any particular aspect of the application. Overdoing the eyes with black liner and dark eyeshadows and not balancing it out with strong lipstick and blush will not look finished. The same is true for lots of blush color and no eyeshadow or lipstick.

Finis

Hopefully, you have followed along beautifully and should be done and looking great. Let me forewarn you that the first time you attempt this it might take you awhile to finish, but be patient. With practice it really can take only seven to twelve minutes.

Four Major Questions to Ask Yourself to Help You Get Started with Your Makeup

1. **How do I normally wear my makeup?** Once you accept how much makeup you're used to wearing you can get a good idea of how much makeup you will feel comfortable putting on. For example, if you are not used to wearing a foundation, then perhaps wearing only a mini-application of foundation will be best. (See Foundation section)

2. **What is a typical or major color in my (seasonal) wardrobe?** This will help you decide which color direction to focus on. Quite frequently you will have both colors in your wardrobe (blue and yellow undertones), which may mean both makeup families are necessary for you. Start with the one you are in most need of. If more blue tones are in your closet, then use those colors to start.

3. **How do I want to look?** This will give you an idea of how intense you should be wearing your makeup. A desire for a more dramatic effect requires more color and defining. A casual, natural looking makeup requires less.

4. **What do I need this makeup for? Work? Social event?** If the makeup is for daytime business, wear a more natural look. If it's for an evening out, and your clothes are more dramatic, then the makeup should be more dramatic.

A Quick Review

Foundation: Smooth over skin with sponge. Use the edge of the sponge that doesn't have makeup on it to buff and remove excess. Foundation blends over the white under the eye and on the eyelid. Avoid placing foundation on or near the jawline.

Brush Strokes: Knock excess powder off of brush before starting, then use short quick motions to apply color.

Contouring: Do before blushing. Use a small blush brush.

Blushing: Avoid blush near eye area. Use a large powder brush.

Lipstick: Line lips first.

Step by Step:

1. Apply white highlighter along inside corner of eye with finger or cotton swab.

2. Apply foundation in dots over central area of face with either fingertips or sponge. BLEND foundation with dry sponge.

3. Eye Design — start with lightest color working darker (optional). Do mascara but don't overdo. If doing eyebrows, do last of all.

4. Contouring — [A] Under cheekbone (optional). [B] Back ⅓ corner of eye into the temple area. [C] Nose contouring (optional).

5. Blushing — on top of contouring (optional) on the cheekbone only, brushing down into the contouring.

6. Line mouth. Apply lipstick (lipbrush optional).

7. Check blending with sponge. No hard lines should be visible whatsoever.

8. Order of application is optional after step two is completed.

Potential Problems

Highlighter problems are caused from using too little or too much white highlighter under the foundation. Too little doesn't give enough coverage, and too much shows through in globs of white.

When using *foundation* be sure to blend evenly, and do not forget the eyelid, especially the outer third (back corner) and next to the eyelashes.

Foundation filling the lines on the face is primarily caused from using too much foundation or too heavy a foundation and then not blending it on thin enough. Use a light weight water-based foundation always and blend well, using a clean edge of your sponge to go over the lines to pick up any excess foundation. Then lightly powder over the line. (Be careful; too much powder will looked caked and thick.)

If the face is lighter or darker than the neck, you will need to follow the color of the neck for your *foundation* color.

Red-brown (blue tones) contour colors should not be used for *nose contour.* Red shading, even when it's muted, on the nose is not attractive. Use tan, taupe or yellow- brown tones only for shading the nose. Red-brown tones though can be used for the temple.

If you have *pale skin,* be sure to blend well to avoid stripes. You can also increase the area of the *temple contour* and *blush* to give the face a bit more color, just be subtle about it; don't overdo. Light skinned women should be using softer tone shadows, blush and lipstick. Darker skin women should be using slightly stronger tones. (Which means during the summer your makeup is going to change.)

When *blush* goes on choppy, it's usually due to one of three things; not enough foundation, poor blending technique with the brush from either over-blending (which wipes off the foundation), or not knocking the excess off the brush and using a blush shade that is too strong or too grainy.

The order for applying the *eye design* is to first do the eyelid color, then the underbrow, followed by the wedge and/or the U-shape crease color and then eyeliner. Temple contour can be applied after or before the eye design. Eyebrows are always done after everything else is finished.

If you are using the *U-shaped design,* be careful not to use too dark a color or it will be difficult to blend. And if you start too dark, the only color left for the back wedge is black.

Pink *eyeshadows* on the lid will make you look like you've been crying.

Don't forget to check for *drippies* after the eye design is complete.

Glasses

When the lens magnifies the eye, make the eye color softer. Make the liner softer and avoid applying a heavy thick coating of mascara.

If the lens demagnifies the eye, increase the color and definition around the eye. But be careful. More color does not mean hard edges. A hard edge with this type of prescription glass will only look like a *small,* hard edge.

Make sure your blush is placed below the edge of the frame of the glasses. You don't want the frame to break up the movement or angle of the blush.

Miscellaneous Information

Judging the Texture of a Powder

One way to judge how a color will go on the skin is by feel. The drier or softer the feel of the powder, the less intense the application. The heavier, wetter, or grainier the feel of the powder the more intense the application. In the first situation, more color will need to be added to build definition. In the latter case, less color is needed to create a design and you can run into trouble with your blending if you use too much.

GENERAL RULE: THE HEAVIER A COLOR GOES ON, THE BETTER IT IS FOR EYELINING. THE SOFTER THE COLOR GOES ON, THE BETTER IT WILL BE FOR SHADING, CONTOUR OR BLUSH.

NOTE: *Try mixing different textures of blushes, eyeshadows, and contour colors (or anything in powder form) with each other or with transluscent powder. You'll double the colors you have to work with by making them softer or darker.*

What's in a Name? Probably Nothing!

When you buy a cosmetic you can be confident that a lipstick will be a lipstick and foundation will be a foundation. However, when you try to buy a color of blush or foundation according to name alone, reality goes right out the door.

The color name of a product reflects image. When you spend $10 on a blush, *Brown* doesn't sound as expensive or as exciting as *St. Tropez Tan.* Foundations may be called *Porcelain,* but what color is porcelain? My porcelain sink at home is white (well, usually white). Choosing by color name is truly frustrating and relatively useless. Choose color according to appearance and how it looks once it's on the face.

Makeup Bags — A Holding Tank

The typical makeup bags that are used to hold cosmetics are completely inefficient. Not only is it impossible to find anything, they are often small and can't hold everything. (Especially when you consider the size of the typical compact you buy. How many mirrors can one person use at a time?) My suggestion is that you purchase a makeup bag that has two sections and a vinyl covering so you can always see what's inside.

Where Do You Put on Your Makeup?

Bathrooms can be the worst place to put on your makeup. If not steamy and damp, then poorly lit. Either invest in good lighting or change locations to the best light source in the house.

Put My Blush Where?

Now, I know some women become skeptical when I use eyeshadow on areas of the face for which the label says it was not intended. The worry is that eyeshadow shouldn't be used for brows, or blush shouldn't be used on the eye or powder liner won't stay on. Retailers would love for you to think that there is a difference and that you can't use a product except for where it is intended. Most powders, whether they're called blush or eyeshadow, contain the same ingredients. Anything that would be harmful to your eyes would be specifically indicated on the package. Worry about color choice, not product type or name.

Choosing a Makeup Artist

I can't recommend anything more than taking the time to get your makeup done and not just once, but several times. Being born female doesn't mean you instinctively know how to put on blush and eyeshadow. It also isn't information handed down from generation to generation. (If anything, our mothers had less information than we do.)

Although getting your makeup done professionally is very important and incredibly helpful, unfortunately the quality of the work you receive can vary greatly. Be prepared to work with the makeup artist as you would your hairdresser. Remember the haircuts you received when you sat down and told the hairdresser to do whatever he/she felt like?

In order to help you select a trained and thoroughly qualified makeup artist, use the following as a checklist:

1. Referrals — how did Dolores turn out when she went? Check with people who've seen the makeup artist you're considering. Don't rely on newspaper ads or the Yellow Pages.

2. How does the makeup artist wear her makeup (if the artist is a woman, that is)? Is it something you'd wish to emulate? Or, something you pray she doesn't do to you?

3. When starting, does the artist say, "What have you been doing with yourself lately?" Rather, you should be asked about your lifestyle. (Do you work in an office? Stay at home with the children? Have you any known allergies to makeup? etc.). A really good question to be asked is "How would you like to see yourself?"

4. Check the artist's background. Where did they study, or who did they train under? Experience isn't everything but it's good information to have when deciding how you're going to spend your money.

The worst that can happen when you see a makeup artist is you won't like the work, and you can always wash it off.

Men and Makeup

This is not a section on men wearing makeup, which is probably the only subject involving makeup I'm not interested in, even a little bit. Rather, I would like to look at men and their attitudes about women wearing makeup. It seems that even though most men couldn't care less about makeup as an industry or art form, they have definite opinions about the subject once it's on the face of someone they're close to. Even though men seem to admire or lust after women who are nicely made up, the truth is, when it comes to the women they actually touch and hold, men generally prefer their women not to wear makeup.

Although on the surface that sounds somewhat chauvinistic, I'm of the opinion that men feeling "their women" wear too much makeup is more an issue of intimacy than one of good old fashioned chauvenism. Think about it for a minute. After spending 10 or 14 minutes neatly applying your eyeshadows, blush and lipstick, how eagerly are you going to want to kiss or hug anyone, more or less a man you're intimate with? Unless, of course, he doesn't mind walking around with half your face on his collar. And what can you say when that happens? "Excuse me, when I hugged you just now, I left part of my cheek on your shirt sleeve." Doesn't that sound intimate?

Now that doesn't mean I'm suggesting you acquiesce and not wear any makeup at all. It's more or less just another way to view the effectiveness or practicality of wearing makeup for whatever reason. And that doesn't necessarily require any action on your part. It's enough to be aware that when you put on makeup, it does create some barriers that aren't there when the face is naked. Perhaps that means you could wear less makeup when you're around the man in your life. Or, if you are wearing full makeup when you're with an intimate other, it could mean you need to give extra attention in other areas like hand holding or walking arm in arm. (Though I'm not convinced much can replace kissing and hugging.)

There's really no answer for this male-female dilemma. Awareness, reality and sympathy is enough to gain from this section. In the long run, when it comes to wearing makeup, always do what is the best for you at any given time, being aware of how makeup can work for or against you.

The Last Comment

Endings are hard for me. I'm not great at saying goodbye in a word or two. It usually takes seventy or eighty. (Although it has always been relatively easy for me to end stories in TV reporting. But that has more to do with the nature of television than with me. In television there's a very specific amount of time that you have to work with and when time's up you have to be done.) When I'm writing, I can just keep on writing and writing and writing. Especially when it comes to makeup, believe me, I can keep on writing. Makeup is a vast subject and there's a lot that can be said about the buying, wearing, and taking off of the stuff. But I want this book to be a beautiful makeup manual, not a remake of *War and Peace.* It has to end sometime, so it might as well end with a discussion about women and their attitudes concerning makeup which follows the previous section nicely.

Professionally and for dress-up I usually wear makeup. All other times I only wear mascara and lipstick. A friend commented once on how she preferred me without all "that stuff" on my face. I asked her what was wrong with the madeup image I presented. (What was I with makeup on; chopped liver?) She said nothing was wrong with the other image, I just look very good without makeup on, ergo I didn't need to wear all that stuff. Her rationale was, if it didn't make me look any "better", why did I bother?

I knew she felt that she was giving me a compliment, telling me I was more attractive naturally. She took for granted that all women wear makeup because it makes them *better.* And she's probably right. Many women feel that way (we're taught to feel that way). But why take the attitude that wearing makeup *makes* you look better? It may make you *feel* better, but that's an emotional response. You can feel attractive anytime; it's up to you, not your makeup. (You may blame it on your makeup, but it's still you and the way you feel.)

I wear makeup because it is a useful tool in my daily life. It can be powerful as well as helpful. It doesn't make me look *more beautiful;* it only makes me look *different.* Looking better and looking different are not synonymous ideas. Now, I know there's a reality to the idea that makeup makes pale, tired, whatever looking skin appear more alive . . . but why adopt that attitude when it creates such a negative self-image and self-imposed trap. Using makeup as a way to be more versatile, more fashionable or powerful is definitely a more freeing attitude than the concept of "with makeup on I'm more beautiful."

Although this attitude of addiction to makeup as a beauty cure-all is hard to overcome, especially given the pressures of advertising and the fashion world, I'm still going to encourage getting rid of it as best I can. Women limiting themselves is not why I wrote this book. Quite the contrary. My goal is to make the business of beauty easier and faster, and to let you know that you're more beautiful than your makeup could ever be.

Suggested Reading

A Consumer's Dictionary of Cosmetic Ingredients, by Ruth Winter, Published by Crown

Any and all issues of the magazine *Drug & Cosmetic Industry*

The Great American Skin Game, by Tony Stabile

Color Me Beautiful, by Carole Jackson

NOTES

NOTES